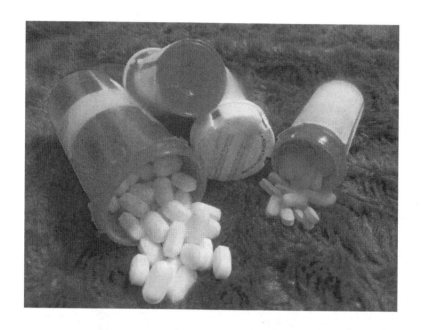

Addiction Recovery Nursing:

An Inside Look

Information for all Nurses

This book is dedicated to The Salvation Army Adult
Recovery Unit in Kansas City. May God bless you always.
It is also dedicated to everyone who has an addiction of any
type.

Amanda, Brittany, Eric and Lauren: I love you.

Bill, thank you for putting up with me all these years.

I love you.

To Ken W., Matt M. and Leeann M. May you see your full
potential and feel the love around you.

Thank you to the God of my understanding, my best friend,
for giving me the courage and endurance to write this much
needed book.

Half of all proceeds from the sale of this book will be given to the
Salvation Army Adult Rehabilitation Center located in Kansas City,
MO.

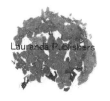

Published by Lauranda Publishers
Overland Park, KS

"I have found that the process of discovering who I really am begins with knowing who I really don't want to be."

(Alcoholics Anonymous, 2001, pp 456-457)

Note to the Reader

The more that I learn about addiction recovery, the more I realize that no one is exempt. Most people have some habit that they have formed in their lives that they want to change. I include myself in this group, so I choose to use the pronoun "we" sometimes in my writing.

As I discuss addiction, I want you to include yourself too. I understand that you may not be addicted to the drugs in this book, but so that you can relate to the recovering addict or the person suffering from substance abuse, please think of something that you want to change in your life. Some of the common substitutes that people have offered me are: shoes, colas, sugary foods, shopping, playing computer games, smoking cigarettes, etc. This is an important part in really understanding the addiction and recovery process.

If you want to see 12-step recovery in action attend an open Alcoholics Anonymous meeting. Open meetings mean that anyone can attend. Remember that these meetings are anonymous. So anything that you see there or hear there should never be repeated outside of the rooms.

The nurse who becomes interested in addiction recovery is a special type of nurse. **We learn to love the addict, but not the addiction.** We learn to see the true person behind the addiction. I feel blessed to be interested and have a passion for this type of nursing.

I really believe that everyone knows at least one person who is or has been addicted to drugs or alcohol. I also believe that this number is increasing every year. Please do not feel that this is something that is far away from you, for it is closer than you think.

Also understand that it takes a long time for the family to heal. They may have spent many years not being able to trust the addict, and now they have a glimmer of hope. If the person begins to use again, that hope is lost again. The family is often hurt, and needs to recover just like the addict. Always remember that this healing can take place with or without the addict.

Many recovery programs are based in a belief and reliance on a Higher Power. Some people choose to call this Higher Power God, while others call Him Jesus, Buddha, etc. **The name is not important**. What is important is the reliance on a power that is not ourselves. It can be anything as long as it is not us. If you choose to use a Higher Power that is used in a religion, then that is fine. Just remember that this Power can be anything as long as it is not you.

Life is about continuously improving oneself. Everyone can learn from many of the recovery programs. Many of them offer a way of living that is pure and true. Many are based in **love and spirituality**. They are based on allowing healing to take place so that we are able to go into the world and heal others. This selfless giving of oneself is what not only keeps the addict clean, but can bring a sense of serenity into a person's life. After all, giving back to others is one of life's golden rules.

Think about some of the greatest contributors to life. Mother Theresa comes to mind. This is what she did. She harnessed the love from God that she received so that she could give it to others. What a blessing.

I hope you find this book useful in your nursing journey. I write all of my books with love. There is no judgement, only understanding. Please feel free to contact me with any suggestions or questions.

May God be with you always.

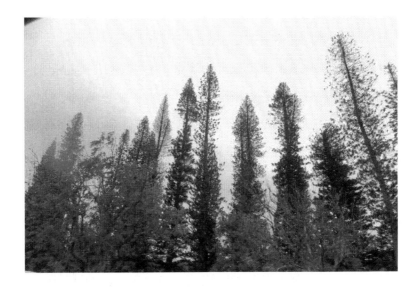

Beauty is all around us, but first we must learn to really see.

Chapter One

Why this Topic?

As I was in the process of writing this book, I had a nurse that I work with ask me why I chose to wrote on this subject. She asked me what I thought I could add to this topic and why it is important for all nurses to understand this complex topic of addiction nursing.

Every year $260,000,000,000 is lost in productivity related to addiction and $52,000,000,000 is spent in the criminal justice system related to addiction and $37,000,000,000 is spent in increased healthcare costs (Lorber, 2013). Only 2% of all money is being used to prevent addiction or treat addiction (Lorber, 2013). In fact, many of our public treatment centers are closing.

In America alone, 2/3 of all families are touched and know someone whose life is being changed by addiction (Lorber, 2013). There are currently 23 million people who are living in long-term recovery, however we still need to reach the other 23 million people who are still suffering from addiction (Lorber, 2013). As healthcare professionals and members of society, I believe that it is our responsibility to do our best to help these people if they want to be helped. In order to accomplish this goal, all healthcare professionals must open their hearts and their minds. We all need to learn about addiction and spread the word across the world.

Substance abuse and addiction is everywhere in our society and we are currently in an opioid abuse crisis. **People do not choose to become addicted**. People do not choose to have their life taken over by substance abuse. Addicts are not people who are weak of will-power either. In fact, many of the recovering addicts that I have met along the way are some of the most intelligent, creative people in the world today.

Medical science has created and proven that many people's brains are predisposed to addiction (Lorber, 2013). This is called the 'Medical Model of Addiction.' We will discuss more of the current models in later chapters. What is important to remember is that **people never set out for the problem to develop.** I have seen many people who at one time were prescribed opioids for chronic or acute pain and have become addicted to the effects of the opioids. They thought that opioids were safe and never considered that they would cross the invisible line of addiction. Most were never educated about this side of pain relief. After weeks of use, they discover the opioid dose must be increased to even touch the pain. When they don't take their medication, they find themselves with more intense pain. They may become nauseous, diaphoretic, anxious, and develop tremors. These are the signs of the body being dependent on the substance. They find that they need to take the drug just to feel normal again. This common situation is proof that the medical model is true.

Drug companies go to great lengths to get doctors to prescribe their drugs. After all, that is what they are in business for, right? It is important for the nurse to completely understand that with the benefit of a medication comes side effects. Be attuned to these effects and before administering a medication, educate the patient.

We are currently experiencing an opioid crisis in the United States. People are finding themselves caught in the spiral of dependence. To give this crisis numbers, I recently read that in 2002 sales of OxyContin rose to over $1.6 billion dollars (Armstrong, 2016). That breaks down to over $133,000,000 a month in sales! The marketers of OxyContin have also found themselves defendants in many cases that stated they misrepresented the drug's addictive qualities (Armstrong, 2016). Is it possible that medical doctors just didn't understand the addictive qualities of this medication?

Regardless of anyone's knowledge of the dependency, the issue continues. Although some of the mixtures are somewhat recent, the issues of dependence and addiction have been in existence since the earliest of times. Using substances to relax probably started when some human, somewhere, decided to chew on some leaf and experienced a sense of euphoria. More people heard about this awesome feeling and tried the plant as well. Soon the village chief found that he/she had a problem on his/her hands. The village was high.

I have also found in my nursing practice that there are quite a few nurses who just don't understand how to care for the alcohol withdrawal patient or who are scared of the person high on a substance. This has to change. Nursing needs to change with the times. If these people are going to come into our practice, then we need to be able to care for them and understand the mechanics of the drugs.

I cannot stress the importance of nurses learning about the information in this book. Medications and drugs are being abused everywhere. **They are in your clinical setting, I guarantee it.** The only way to help our patients with these problems is to learn about addiction and recovery. We need to talk about it and destroy any negative social stigma that is present in our society. No one who wants help should ever have to suffer. People need to be educated about addiction and dependence. People deserve our help. Worldwide there are over 19 million nurses (based on 2011 World Health Organization statistics) (Learning Nurse, 2013). In America alone, there are over 5 million nurses (Learning Nurse, 2013). With numbers like this, it is obvious why nurses are the profession that can reach the masses.

Throughout this book, I will ask you to connect with me through self-reflection. All I ask is that you be honest with your answers. I promise, that if you are able to be honest, you will gain insight into yourself and your views. Writing will also help you to engage in the subject. Fair enough?

If you have decided that the online version of this book is the way to go, then please have a notebook that you can not only take notes in, but you can also journal your answers to my questions. This book is meant to be interactive in nature.

This book is filled with information. I have covered the information that I believe is useful. I want you to understand that addiction recovery is a very complex topic. There are many academic arguments pertaining to the topic. I may bring up a few of these arguments, however solving the addiction problem is not the purpose of this book. The purpose of this book **is to provide all nurses with a basic understanding of drug/alcohol addiction and recovery.**

Please answer the following question: What purpose does learning about addiction recovery serve you in your nursing practice?

Words of Recovery:

"...there is much work to do,

and none of us can do it

standing still."

(Alcoholics Anonymous, 2001, p 534)

Part One

Let's Talk about Addiction

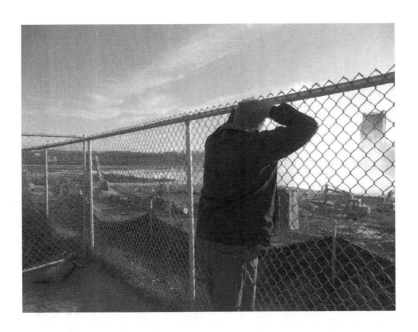

Words of Recovery:

"The dream world has been replaced by a great sense of purpose,"

(Alcoholics Anonymous, 2001, p 130)

Chapter Two

Addiction:

Some Basic Facts

People do not set out to become addicts. They start to use the drug or medication for a purpose. Maybe it is to relieve pain or to be social. As they continue to use, they cross a line. Crossing this line means that the body and mind have adjusted to having this chemical present. When this chemical is not present, an intense craving takes place which often leads the person to use again. The person often finds that they must use the drug to even feel **normal.**

Many people are able to relate to this craving when I mention caffeine. People do not mean to get addicted to caffeine. I love my diet colas, and my husband loves coffee. When I do not have a diet cola, I begin to get a headache and my body asks for it. As soon as I drink one, the headache goes away and I feel normal again. Addiction to caffeine is acceptable in our society, however caffeine is also a stimulant drug which has effects on our body and mind.

When we are able to say, "I have a habit or addiction," addiction recovery calls this **awareness**. Let's be honest, many people are aware that they have problems, but they are comfortable with them. They may even justify the habit. I can say that caffeine helps me to wake up! Being aware of an issue, **is simply being aware**. It does not mean that the person wants to take the steps to change.

Many addicts are aware that they have a problem. They may even be aware that the problem is **causing issues in their lives**. They may even say, "So what?" I mention this because I don't want anyone to ever equate **awareness** with **recovery**. **Awareness is simply awareness**. It will lead to action, but the action could be using.

Logic and addiction are actually related, but some people cannot imagine their life without their drug of choice. Think about this: If something makes you feel kind of normal when you use it, how fast would you be to give it up? How fast would you give it up if when you didn't use it, you felt terrible? This is the logic of addiction and the great fact.

People may know that they need to quit, and they may have figured out that when they use substances, it causes problems in their life, however this does not mean that they are going to quit. Once the addiction line is crossed, stopping is painful and the pull of continuing the habit is very strong. Stopping often becomes painful and mentally confusing. At least for a short time.

> **The pull of any addiction is very strong and it is important to remember that the person has most likely been practicing the habit for a long time. The body has become used to the substance and the mind has learned how to function with the substance present.**

Addiction can lead the addict into many dark places. Places that others may not understand. The need to the drug may be so strong that the addict becomes willing to do anything to satisfy the craving. This is a scary fact of addiction. **Many addicts do things that they never thought they would do in order to obtain their drug.**

I also want to explain that when it comes to drug or alcohol addiction, people often have a **drug of choice**. This is the substance that they crave the most. They may use other substances, but the drug of choice is like their cherry on the top of their addiction cake.

What is an Addict?

What is an **addict**? For the purpose of this book, we are going to define an addict as **someone who has crossed the line with a habit.** This person's body and mind craves the chemical. There is no judgement on this person as the process that happens within the human body is a biological one that probably has helped us survive decades. Our minds also adjust to the habit. The addict reaches a point where he/she cannot imagine life without the habit.

Figure 2.1 Crossing the Addiction Line.

Preaddiction	THE ADDICTION LINE	ADDICTION
Can partake in the action with no consequences.	Body and mind learn to adapt to haveing the chemical present. Often use more frequently.	Crave the chemical. Find functioning without the chemical very difficult.

Why Do People Become Addicts?

There are many models that try to define why people become addicted to substances. Some of these models are based on biology, while others are based in psychology. In this chapter I will touch on a few of the models.

The Medical Model

The medical model has been proven time and time again. The medical model states that as time and use continues, the body physiologically craves the drug and greater amounts are needed to achieve the desired effect (Dossey and Keegan, 2013). When the drug is not present in the body, our bodies actually crave the substance. This is because the mind rewires itself to accommodate the substance.

Many drugs cause an increase in dopamine at the synapses in the brain. When our brains sense the increase of dopamine, it begins to destroy receptors. As the receptors are destroyed, it takes an increase of the substance to feel any effect. As the substance is increased, more receptors die. This causes the cycle to continue. When the person does not have the substance present, he/she feels terrible as the constant level of dopamine has been decreased because of the decrease in receptors. This is why the person finds that they need to use to even feel normal.

Mentally, dopamine regulates our movements, emotions, motivation, pleasure, and cognition (Dossey and Keegan, 2013, p 542). A decrease in dopamine can cause a person to have mental effects, however withdrawal of the drug also causes physical effects. Many of the common physical effects include tremors, nausea, chills, hallucinations, and other 'flu-like' symptoms. When we combine all of these feelings, is there any question why abuse continues medically?

The bottom line is that some drugs make us feel better, at least at first. As the use continues, our bodies and mind change to accommodate the effects. When we stop, we feel terrible. This is how the drugs work.

Why is Addiction Considered a Disease?

Addiction is considered a disease because it progresses. If it is not treated, then most people will die from it. That is the plain and simple truth of it. We know that the addict will crave more and more of the substance. Even when the addict quits, it is thought that they never recover, but are always in the process of recovery. If an addict could recover, that would mean that a person who was once an alcoholic could have just one drink and be satisfied. That is usually not the case once the line is crossed. One drink reactivates the craving and the process starts over again. **The disease can be placed in remission, but never cured.** Remission is obtained by not using and recovering.

Figure 2.2 Example of the Medical Model

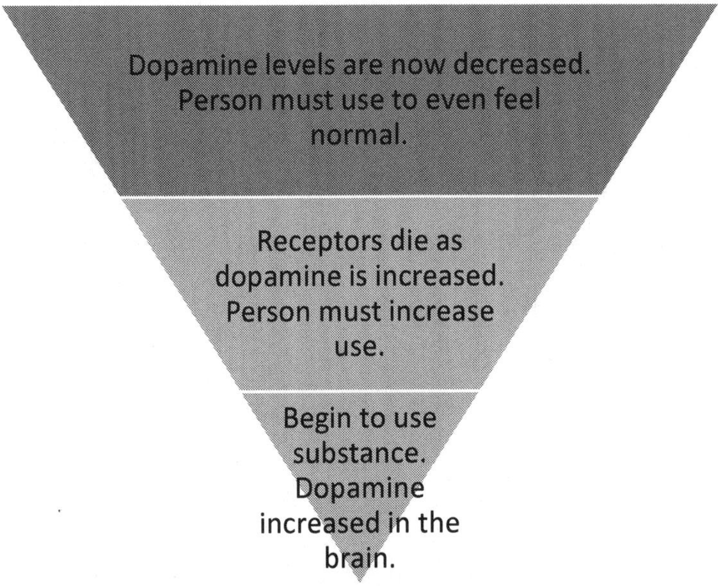

Dopamine levels are now decreased. Person must use to even feel normal.

Receptors die as dopamine is increased. Person must increase use.

Begin to use substance. Dopamine increased in the brain.

The Genetic Disease Model

Addiction has been found to run in families. This is tied to genetics. Adopted children have been studied to see if the disease continues in the family tree even if the children are raised in a nonalcoholic home (Dossey and Keegan, 2013). Researchers have shown that these children show a three times greater incidence of alcoholism even when raised in an alternative environment (Dossey and Keegan, 2013).

Since the Human Genome Project, the field of epigenetics has been growing. Through various studies in this field, researcher have discovered important information about addiction. The Genetic Disease Model states that the family link is most likely biochemical in nature (Dossey and Keegan, 2013). This means that the amount of chemicals or the amount of receptors in our brain are predetermined through heredity. When the chemical increases the amount of the neurotransmitter, we finally feel okay. Perhaps increased frequency of substance abuse through time causes adaptation which results in familial changes in genetic expression (Dossey and Keegan, 2013).

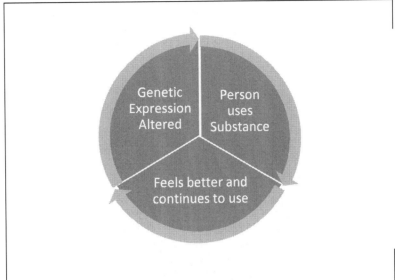

Figure 2.3 Genetic Disease Model

The Cultural Model

The cultural model states that our culture is based on immediate gratification and we are taught to seek answers outside of ourselves (Dossey and Keegan, 2013). We are taught that "there is a pill for every ill," (Dossey and Keegan, 2013, p. 544). This message is taught to us through the media (Dossey and Keegan, 2013).

In 2015 the United States pharmaceutical industry spent over $5.2 billion dollars on just direct advertising to consumers (ProCon.org,2016). These are the ads that we often see on commercials or in the paper. They are the ads that talk directly to the non-medical community. These ads focus on both prescription and over-the-counter (OTC) medications. Although many of these advertisements inform consumers, they also may misinform them as well (ProCon.org, 2016).

Although the Food and Drug Administration (FDA) monitors these advertisements, 74% of physicians stated that these advertisements overemphasize the benefits of the drugs (ProCon.org, 2016). Drug-related emergency room visits also increased 81% from 2004 to 2009 (2.5 million to 4.6 million) (Dossey and Keegan, 2013, p. 544). Nonmedical use of pharmaceuticals increased 98.4% during this time period as well (Dossey and Keegan, 2013, p 544).

Figure 2.4 the Cultural Model of Abuse

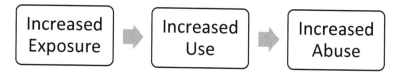

Psychosexual, Psychoanalytic Model

Freud believed that addiction was based on the oral phase of the psychosexual stages of development (Dossey and Keegan, 2013). When an infant's needs are unmet at this stage, the person becomes orally fixated and seeks oral gratification (Dossey and Keegan, 2013). As a result of the unmet oral needs, emotional growth is stopped as well (Dossey and Keegan, 2013, p 543). Freud believed that the addict is actually trying to fulfill this unmet need through using.

Character Defect Model of Alcoholics Anonymous

Alcoholics Anonymous (AA) discusses character defects as a potential cause for abuse (Dossey and Keegan, 2013). This character defect can be a single issue, however it is more commonly multiple issues or experiences that have been unresolved. These character defects may be attributable to the difficulty in making changes in one's life (Dossey and Keegan, 2013).

Transpersonal Intoxication Model

The final model that we will discuss in this book is the Transpersonal Intoxication Model. This model states that people who become addicted to substances do so because they are trying to break free of a limited sense of self (Dossey and Keegan, 2013). These people are trying to gain additional experiences and expand their minds through expanded states of awareness.

This state of expansion has been noted in the past by musicians and artists. This mode of thinking was introduced in the 1960's and still exists in part. At first the artist may find that the drug expands their creativity, however with continued use, the creativity is reliant upon the use of the drug (Dossey and Keegan, 2013).

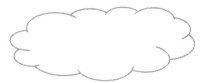

It should be noted that the models that have been listed are only a partial list of the theories of addiction. There are many others. Studies continue into the cause of addiction because if we figure out what causes it, perhaps we can cure it. Perhaps there is no one cure, but rather multiple cures. Perhaps one theory does not ring true for everyone, but a combination of theories are needed.

A Note to Nurses on Addiction

This book is written for nurses. As you read through these pages, please do not think that the people who use these drugs are far away from you. That is what I thought for a long time. I thought that heroin was a problem in the inner cities, not in the suburban hospitals! Surely, I would never see an 80 year old patient who uses these drugs! I was wrong. People who have substance abuse problems and addiction are everywhere. Some patients are just better at hiding their use or addiction better than others.

As you obtain the history on your patients, do not be nervous to ask about drug or alcohol use/abuse. There are many reputable addiction questionnaires available. If your facility incorporates these scales into the admission process, make sure that you ask these questions to your patients. Ask the question, pause, and let them answer. *Maybe they will tell you the truth.*

Learning about addiction recovery nursing is not an alienated specialty. Studying addiction recovery in nursing goes hand in hand with learning about pain management because some addictions are started as a result of the person trying to manage pain. Many addiction recovery nurses also find it useful to learn about alternative medicine. Eastern and other non-Western therapies have been helpful to humans for thousands of years and has proven useful to many people.

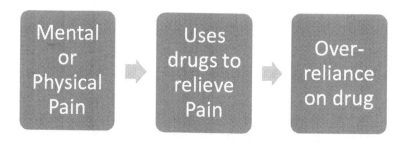

It is also important for the addiction recovery nurse to learn about psychological issues such as depression and anxiety, as these also seem to be prevalent in people who suffer from addiction. It is important to note that some doctors are hesitant to prescribe new psychological medications to newly recovery addicts for the first six months of recovery. The chemicals in the brain are altered by the frequent use of the substance. It takes time for the body and the brain to heal.

Addiction can happen to anyone and many addicts are quite intelligent people who have made harmful decisions. The cycle begins and then continues until the "high" no longer is pleasant, however the addict physically and mentally needs the drug. In fact, many active addicts cannot imagine their life without their drug of choice.

Is the addict at fault? Well, the decision to use is always a decision, but no one sets off with the goal of becoming an addict. Maybe people do not understand how easily a person can become addicted. Perhaps the medical community needs to join together and continue to educate. This education must occur within our medical community and within the communities that we live. We must be aware of the problem and understand that we are the ones that have the ability to educate. The best place to stop an addiction is before it ever begins.

Programs that educate and keep people from beginning to use are one of the best places to start this education. In community health nursing we call this "primary prevention." Primary prevention is when we stop the disease before it ever has a chance to occur.

As nurses educate in the community and researchers try to uncover why some people become addicts, we can only wonder. Perhaps there is something different in the wiring of the brain that predisposes some people to a lifetime of being confronted with addictive behavior or maybe anyone can become addicted. Why can one person drink an alcoholic beverage and have no light bulb go off, while other people have a major light bulb go off that tells them that this is the answer that they have been searching for? Why do some people find their addiction early in life, while others discover it later in life? How do people chose their drug of choice?

Self-Reflection:

When I think of addiction, I think of:

(Finish this sentence) People who are addicted to drugs and/or alcohol are _____.

I want to learn about:

Words of Recovery:

"Attendees share ideas with only one purpose in mind- to help one another,"

(SMART recovery, 2010)

Chapter Three
Society's View

The concept of addiction has concerned people since the earliest of times. Fermented beverages were known to exist in China since 7000 B.C.E. and in India since 3000 to 2000 B.C.E. (Drugfreeworld.org, 2006-2016). In 2700 B.C.E it is known that the Babylonians worshiped the wine (fermentation) goddess, Suduri (Drugfreeworld.org, 2006-2016). Although the substances that were used in the creation of the drinks differed, the end-effect was the same.

The effect of opium was understood and the flower cultivated since at least 3400 B.C.E. in lower Mesopotamia (Atlantic Monthly Group, 2016). Known as the "Joy Plant" it was shared with the Assyrians and Egyptians (Atlantic Monthly Group, 2016). The plant was later used by Hippocrates around 460-357 B.C.E. for its apparent medicinal purposes (Atlantic Monthly Group, 2016).

It appears that the use of many of these substances were accepted in society, however the overuse was frowned upon. Even the Old Testament and the New Testament discusses wine and drunkards. It addresses the concept that man should not get drunk with wine for this action will interfere with the ability to enter Heaven (Open Bible, 2016). So the consumption of wine is acceptable, it is the overconsumption that is frowned upon.

America has accepted the use of many mind altering substances for medicinal use (Casey, 1978). Alcohol has seen acceptance as well as rejection. Abstentionist outcries around Civil War years may have contributed to the prohibition (Casey, 1978). On an 18th century pamphlet, the use of any drink "which is liable to steal away a man's senses and render him foolish, irascible, uncontrollable and dangerous," was warned against (Casey, 1978).

Many of the substances that are abused today, were once legal and used acceptably. At one time in American history, opium dens were present throughout the west coast (Casey, 1978). As one substance would be lawed illegal, then the people would search for other alternative ways to reach a high. This is the trend throughout time.

Throughout time, there has always been extremist groups. Some groups state that the use of any substance is bad, while other groups state that the people should have the right to decide. The middle ground states that use of most legal substances are okay, but society suffers once the addiction line is crossed. Once the addiction line is crossed, society frowns on the use of any substance. Through a fear of being alienated, many people suffered in silence.

Perhaps society frowns upon addiction through a sense of fear, Fear of the known and the unknown. Maybe the fear is a reflection of our own vulnerability. Society realizes that this epidemic can effect anyone at any time.

Once the physical and mental effects of addiction were noted, many members of society worked to find a cure or treatment (Patterson, 2016). Medical science was baffled by addiction. There were no recovery houses and many addicts spent time in the mental hospitals which did not seem to help. Addicts often found themselves the subjects of cruel medical practices like lobotomies. Addiction was treated as a moral weakness, and was often treated as an illness or as a criminal offense (Patterson, 2016).

Benjamin Rush, one of the Founding Fathers of America, "was one of the first to believe that alcoholism was not a matter of personal willpower but rather due to the alcohol itself," (Patterson, 2016). Rush was the first person to fight for the concept that alcoholism was in fact, a disease (Patterson, 2016).

It was not until 1864 that the New York State Inebriate Asylum was opened (Patterson, 2016). This hospital's main purpose was to treat alcoholics and considered alcoholism a mental health condition. As a result of public concern, more community assistance began to develop.

In spite of all of the efforts, a cure was not in sight. Religious groups often stated that addiction was indeed a disease of the spirit and prayed feverously for the addict. As an attempt to help addicts recover, many community sobriety groups began to appear. One of the largest of these groups was the Oxford Group. This group was founded by Frank Buchman.

After Frank had a spiritual experience, he founded an evangelical group in Oxford University in England (Sacred Connections, 2009). The movement was based on simple principles and spread worldwide over the next few decades (Sacred Connections, 2009). The movement believed in "absolute surrender, guidance by the Holy Spirit, sharing in fellowship, life changing faith and prayer while aiming for absolute Love, Purity, Honesty and Unselfishness (Sacred Connections, 2009). The movement also practiced the principles of the 5 C's: "confidence, confession, conviction, conversion and continuance," (Sacred Connections, 2009). In 1928 the group became known as the Oxford Group (Sacred Connections, 2009). The Oxford Group believed they had a remedy for many of life's ills, including addiction.

The principles of the Oxford Group pertaining to addiction were described as admitting being licked, getting honest with ourselves, talking over things with another, making amends to anyone harmed along the way, carrying the message with no thought of reward and praying to whatever God we though there was (Sacred Connections, 2009). Many people were helped through the efforts of this group and it was the seed that created the tree of Alcoholics Anonymous.

Another movement in history is known as the Temperance Movement. This movement occurred in the 19th and early 20th century and was fueled by women who had become tired of their men drinking (Encyclopedia Britannica, 2016). The movement promoted moderation and encouraged abstinence (Encyclopedia Britannica, 2016). The movement grew through the churches and the concepts became the subject of education in society (Encyclopedia Britannica, 2016). Susan B. Anthony was a famous member of the Temperance Movement (Encyclopedia Britannica, 2016). This movement displays the view that moderation of consumption is okay, but overindulgence should be prohibited.

Another movement that influenced the United States was Prohibition that lasted from 1920 to 1933. Although the law prohibited the use, importation, transportation, and sale of alcoholic products, it did not change society's consumption pattern. Although it fought for abstinence, it did not solve the addiction problem. It did confirm mainstream society's acceptance of alcohol.

The medical view has developed in recent years. Addiction is becoming a science. Medical science is learning that people who have addictive personalities, may actually be hard-wired differently. Scientists are learning that every drug (including alcohol) releases specific neurotransmitters in the brain as it causes chemical reactions. Do you think this is true or do we all have the capacity to become addicted?

Current views appear to be mixed. Some people believe that addiction is a disease, while others think that it can be controlled by the abuser. Acceptance of different substances also depends on legality and fear. It seems that moderate use of legal substances is accepted in modern society, while abuse or use of illegal substances is frowned upon.

A Little More Neuroscience

It is actually amazing to think how far neuroscience has come even in the last few years. When I took my first neuroscience class in the 1990's, scientists had only identified a few of the chemicals in the brain. Now, we have identified many chemicals and those chemicals have variations! It is incredible how far we have come. I can't wait to see what the future holds.

We have learned that when we are happy, our brain releases chemicals that make us happy, and when we are sad, different chemical changes in the brain take place. Physical activity can also release chemicals. I think that we are safe to say that every thought we have and every physical activity we participate in releases a chemical or two. If everything that our brain processes is completed through chemicals, then neuroscience has learned that it is possible to change these chemicals for our advantage.

Take a minute to think about SSRI's. These medications change the amount of serotonin that is exchanged between our synapses. Drugs like morphine and heroin, increase the amount of dopamine in these synapses. Alcohol affects our GABA receptors. Every drug, whether legal or illegal, effects our bodies in some way. Some drugs, are even able to effect the chemicals in our brain.

Scientists seem to be constantly working on ways to ease the recovery process. They are busy in the laboratories trying to make pills that can block the effects on the neurotransmitters that are created through the use of the substance.

Do you think this will stop the addict from using?

Part II

Recovery

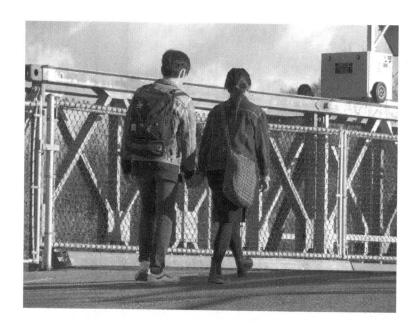

Words of Recovery:

I am not sure why it happened, but I know that it was a miracle of sorts.

Chapter Four

Nursing Care

The Acute Phase of Recovery

A recovery book and a Bible should be in the side table drawer in every hospital. This is how common this problem is.

In 2013 it was estimated that over 22.7 million people in the United States alone needed treatment for an alcohol or drug abuse problem (Rundio & Lorman, 2015). Although alcohol is still considered the number one drug of choice in the United States, cannabis is slowly closing in (Rundio & Lorman, 2015). In 2007 The National Drug Intelligence Center reported that the cost of illicit drug use in the United States cost more than 193 billion dollars (National Drug Intelligence Center, 2012). Heroin, marijuana, methamphetamines and prescription drug abuse were found to be on the serious incline among the youth in the United States (National Drug Intelligence Center, 2012). Although these reports are only available through archives from the Department of Justice, these numbers have most likely only increased. It is impossible to deny the impact that these substances have on America's health.

When people decide to recover, care for the newly **recovering addict is complex**. Nurses need to have a working knowledge of this process. Although the initial acute care relies on supportive treatments, later treatment must involve a complete physical assessment, spiritual assessment, psychosocial assessment, social assessment and labs. It should also include questions that can help to identify any suicidal ideations that may be present (Rundio & Lorman, 2015).

Many early recovering addicts are malnourished and often quite dehydrated. It is important to run IV fluids in the acute phases of recovery and then later the nurse must encourage the person to eat a well-balanced diet and drink plenty of water. This may not be possible right away, but in time the appetite will most likely increase. All addicts should be screened for STD's, including HIV. Hep C tests should also be run.

If your patient is on alcohol withdrawal, then they should be placed on the Clinical Institute Withdrawal Assessment for Alcohol (CIWA) protocol. This protocol was created by the Centre for Addiction and Mental Health (CAMH, 2001). It asks the nurse to rate 10 withdrawal signs. Some of these signs are Nausea and vomiting, anxiety, sweats, visual disturbances, etc. (CAMH, 2001). The higher that a patient scores, the more intense the withdrawal symptoms are. Once a score is obtained, hospital protocol becomes involved.

Hospital protocol varies. Some protocols say that if the score is above 15, then the person should go to the ICU for more intense treatment, while other protocols are okay with this number. Usually if the score is above 8, then the person is treated with a benzodiazepine, such as lorazepam or diazapam. If you treat the person, then you must reassess on a continual basis. Some hospitals state that you should reassess within one hour. I am a firm believer that if you believe that the withdrawal is intense enough to treat, then you better keep a close eye on them. They also earn a room right across from the nurses' station in my practice. Alcohol withdrawal can kill. Take withdrawal symptoms seriously.

When you get a patient who is on an alcohol withdrawal protocol, please do not be afraid. I have seen so many nurses become so timid when dealing with these patients. This is not to say that you do not need to be careful. Take all precautions and protect yourself as you care for them. This is important for everyone involved. It is also important that you treat them with the appropriate amount of medication as they are going through the withdrawal process.

Follow the recommendations on the second page of the scale. In other words, take the sheet with you and explain what you are doing to the patient (CAMH, 2001). Ask the patient if they have any questions and tell them that you will be frequently monitoring them (CAMH, 2001). Inform the patient what their current score is if you think that they will benefit from hearing the result (CAMH, 2001).

Many hospitals do not use them, however there are also many opioid withdrawal scales used in addiction medicine. These scales are often used before methadone or other medicinal treatment is initiated (Wesson & Ling, 2003). One of these scales is called the Clinical Opiate Withdrawal Scale. It is also known as COWS, however I would be hesitant to call it that in a clinical setting. This scale is very similar to the CIWA scale, although it looks for symptoms that are present in opioid withdrawal patients. Some of these symptoms have been defined as yawning, rhinorrhea, vomiting, muscle twitches, restlessness, piloerection, abdominal cramps, tremors, etc. (Wesson & Ling, 2001). It is important for all nurses to learn the signs and symptoms of opioid withdrawal. This is because the patient who is in withdrawal may not always identify the lack of opioids as the cause. You may have a patient that is displaying all of the signs and symptoms, however expensive tests are being run because opioid withdrawal is not being considered.

It is also important to note that there are many opiate withdrawal scales. The first scale used was created by Handlesman through the Federal Addiction Research Center in Lexington, Kentucky in 1937 (Wesson & Ling, 2003). C.K. Handlesman was a medical doctor that studied addiction beginning in the 1930's. His scale measures the degree of opiate withdrawal either by the hour or the day (Wesson & Ling, 2003). It has a 15 point consideration and measures many of the same withdrawal signs that are measured above (Wesson & Ling, 2003). Added withdrawal signs are fever, elevated morning systolic blood pressure, hyperpnea and weight loss (Wesson & Ling, 2003). It is important to note that Himmelsbach's scale is primarily objective in nature and also serves as the base model for later scales (Wesson & Ling, 2003).

The next scale that was developed in the Federal Addiction Research Center was the Opiate Withdrawal Subjective Experience (OPW) scale in the 1960's (Wesson & Ling, 2003). This 550 item questionnaire is not really useful in clinical practice, however it could potentially be used in research. What patient would want to answer 550 questions?

Many other scales have been developed that can assist in rating opioid withdrawal. The COWS scale is the scale that is currently recommended for clinical use as it can be used in a variety of settings and is not time consuming (Wesson & Ling, 2003). It is also useful in many different instances.

A Cannabis Withdrawal Scale (CWS) is also in existence (Allsop, Copeland, Fu & Budney, 2011). This scale was originally tested in a study that included 49 participants over a two week abstinence (Allsop et al, 2011). The researchers tested the volunteer participants after one week of abstinence and then again at two weeks abstinence (Allsop et al, 2011). Allsop et al (2011) reported that the most valid withdrawal symptom was nightmares/strange dreams, however these did not seem to cause the subjects much distress. Other withdrawal symptoms that were reported as troublesome to the participants were angry outbursts and trouble falling to sleep (Allsop et al, 2011).

As a note: If you are interested in recovery nursing, there is a recovery nurse certification that is offered by the International Nurses Society on Addiction (INTNSA). Certifications are always a great asset to any nurse and the information that one needs to learn to sit for this exam is very interesting. It involves history, treatment plans, diagnosing, and risk reduction.

There are many scales available that can rate a person's addiction to a substance or activity. Many of these scales have been proven valid and serve as a great point to start a discussion. The most reliable source is when the patient admits he/she has a problem.

FYI:

It is important to remember that the majority of standard drug screens in the acute care setting only test for THC, PCP, Opiates, cocaine, alcohol (ethanol and methanol), amphetamines, barbiturates, methadone and benzodiazepines. If the person is on another substance that is not included on the toxicity screen, then the only way that the acute care team can identify the substance is if the patient can identify it.

Words of Recovery:

"It wasn't easy, and it has never been easy, but it gets so much better."

(Alcoholics Anonymous, 2001, p 288)

Chapter Five

Recovery Programs

First, let me say that there are so many recovery programs that I could not possibly cover them in this book. Each seem to have a different twist and not all of them are right for everyone. It is important for the person who wants to recover to decide on the program that he/she feels will be most beneficial to him/her. Sometimes a person must try more than one program before success is achieved. Some of the programs are Higher Power driven and some are not.

Recovery programs can be inpatient or outpatient. The best treatment really depends on the person. Many things need to be considered before the right rehabilitation program is selected. Some of these factors are cost and insurance, inpatient or outpatient, life responsibilities, living situation, beliefs, and the program itself. Recovery is not one size fits all, but with willingness and desire, recovery is possible. It is also important to note that many private recovery programs may advertise locally, but actually are located in areas like California and Florida. Location sometimes matters to people.

Twelve-step programs such as Alcoholics Anonymous are probably the most popular. They are free to attend. Because of their importance in recovery, I will discuss that program in another chapter. I am including a partial list of some recovery organizations for reference.

Partial List of Recovery Organizations (Not 12-Step Organizations)

SMART Recovery
Self-Management and Recovery Training
On-line and meetings, books available
http://www.smartrecovery.org/

16 Steps for Discovery and Empowerment
http://charlottekasl.com/16-step-program/

Celebrate Recovery
Christ based recovery
Meetings, events, books, videos
http://www.celebraterecovery.com/

Rational Recovery
https://rational.org/index.php?id=1

MM: Moderation Management
Meetings, literature, blogs
Believes in self-control and moderation
http://moderation.org/

Addiction Survivors.org
On line forums
http://www.addictionsurvivors.org/

HAMS: Harm Reduction Network
Based on 17 optional elements
http://hams.cc/

LifeRing Secular Recovery
Books, meetings, blogs
http://lifering.org/

Alcoholics for Christ
Meetings
http://www.alcoholicsforchrist.com/

Buddhist Recovery Network
Meetings, events and literature
http://www.buddhistrecovery.org/

Addiction Alternatives
http://addictionalternatives.com/

Secular Organizations for Sobriety (SOS)
http://www.sossobriety.org/

Exposure Response Prevention (ERP)
Believes in exposing the addict to the substance of choice
and desensitizing the craving.
http://www.killthecraving.com/

Dual Recovery Anonymous
Substance abuse plus mental disorder
http://www.draonline.org/

Recovery Chatrooms
Free, but encourage donations
Chat rooms
http://www.recoverychat.com/

Daily Strength
Online
https://www.dailystrength.org/categories/Addiction_Recov
ery

As I said, this is just a partial list of the self-help
recovery groups available to your patients. Some people
combine programs. This is usually okay as long as the
person does not get confused and their method is working
for them. The important thigs to remember is that there is
no one right way to stop an addiction.

In-patient programs differ in many ways. The type of treatment depends greatly on the individual needs, insurance coverage and cost. All treatment facilities are either non-profit or for-profit. Some are run on contributions while others include work therapy. Whatever center is agreed on, the plan of care should comply with the Center for Substance Abuse Treatment (Rundio & Lorman, 2015). This organization works through the Substance Abuse and Mental Health Services Asociation (SAMHSA) "improve access, reduce barriers, and promote high quality, effective treatment and recovery services," (SAMHSA, 2016). Bringing down the barriers to treatment and recovery is important. In 2013, only 7.9% of the American population were able to get treatment for their addiction (Rundio & Lorman, 2015). This needs to change.

Official treatment program lengths vary. Some last for 21 days, while others last for a year. Although many people find it difficult to stop their life for this period of time, it is important to remind them that without this treatment, they may not have a life to come back to. Recovery is their main priority.

Spiritual approaches to addiction have brought about controversy with some social workers, however these programs are probably the most commonly used recovery programs (Dossett, 2013). Project MATCH, which took place in the United States in the 1990's, compared the effectiveness of 12-step spiritually based programs with cognitive behavioral coping skills therapy and motivational enhancement therapy (Dossett, 2013). This study showed that 12-step programs are at least as effective in treatment as the other academically based treatment programs (Dossett, 2013).

Words of recovery:

Sometimes the best thing that we can do for our recovery is to get out of our own way.

-Anonymous

Chapter Six

Recovery through the 12-Steps

As we explore recovery, we will concentrate on those programs of recovery that are spiritually based. The largest worldwide program is Alcoholics Anonymous (AA). AA is present in over 170 countries and has over 2 million members around the world (AA Central Service, 2016). Of course, since membership in the organization is anonymous, there is no way to achieve an exact count of the total members. This number is only an estimate.

The concepts that are used in the AA program have led to the birth of many additional addiction recovery organizations. Some of these are Cocaine Anonymous, Narcotics Anonymous, Crystal Meth Anonymous, Marijuana Anonymous, etc. If there is one recovery program that has worked through out the years, it is AA. Perhaps it is because membership to any of these organizations is free, and involves one recovering alcoholic talking to another. The program involves accountability and is based on togetherness. A basic understanding of the concepts of AA are important for any nurse interested in addiction recovery.

Twelve step programs are based on the recovering addicts working through 12 spiritually based steps. These steps involve admitting there is a problem, asking a Higher Power for help, acknowledging one's mistakes, asking forgiveness, and helping others. The recovering addict continues through the steps throughout the recovery process.

One of the most chosen recovery programs available is Alcoholics Anonymous (AA) (Dossett, 2013). AA members work very hard to help all healthcare professionals effectively deal with problem drinkers (Alcoholics Anonymous, 2016). If you have a patient who wishes to recover, it is always possible for the nurse to give the patient the number to the closest AA central office. Often times, members will come and visit those people wishing to recover while they are in the hospital. It is important to note that AA uses a spiritual approach in addressing the recovery process, however it does not align itself with any other organization (Alcoholics Anonymous, 2016). AA also offers a free on-line newsletter for all

Let's Explore Some Concepts of Recovery

There are many addiction recovery programs and many theories on how to recover. Some of these programs and models introduce the concept of a **Higher Power**. Many people ask, "What is a Higher Power and why should this matter?" **A Higher Power is something that is greater than ourselves.** It can be anything, as long as it is not the habit that we are trying to change, and not ourselves. It is a Power that the addict will hopefully begin to rely on. It is not necessarily about organized religion, although that is where some recovering addicts find their Higher Power. It is about a connection with the Power of the Universe. Many call this Higher Power, "God." It is interesting that when Bill W. wrote the 12 steps and the members saw that God was mentioned quite a few times, they became concerned. Do not get caught up in the details.

Through intense souls searching, and talking with other spiritual people, the recovering addict becomes willing to admit that he/she cannot recover on his/her own and that a greater power is needed.

The pull of addiction can be quite intense. In fact, at times it is so intense, that many spiritually based recovery programs encourage the recovering addict to give their addiction and all of their problems to a Higher Power. Talking about the craving with another recovering alcoholic is also vital. This action is called **surrender. Surrender in recovery is a confirmation that help is needed.** It is a new feeling for many recovering addict. It means that the fight is over for this moment. When humans are able to admit their feelings, it is though the power of the feeling lessons.

It is important for the recovering addict to remember that "surrender" is an action verb and the recovering addict must learn to surrender his/her will continuously (Alcoholics Anonymous, 2016). **Recovery in 12-step programs is about surrendering to a Higher Power.**

Turn your problems over to a Higher Power.

Healing from any addiction takes time and dedication. It takes turning one's will over to that Higher Power and admitting that He knows more than we do. As humans, we realize that we are not perfect and we do not have all of the answers.

About Perfection

A few years ago, my mom was diagnosed with uterine cancer. Went I went to be with her, I felt like I needed to have all of the answers. After all, I am a nurse. I was very hard on myself.

One day, a fellow nurse came up to me and said, "I give you permission to be a daughter today." I asked her what she meant by that. She explained to me that even though I was a nurse, this person in front of me was my Mom. I was a daughter first.

I learned to put down my nurse hat at that moment and enjoy being a daughter. I placed my confidence in my fellow nurses and the doctor as I realized that God had everything in control. I was able to hold my Mom's hand through the recovery process and be her daughter. I did not have to be perfect.

Emotions and Recovery

Feeling emotions is an important concept when we discuss recovery. Many addicts have a hard time dealing with emotions. Perhaps they were not permitted to show them while they were growing up, and they never learned what they were as a result. What if any time you were happy, sad, or mad, you were beat? What if anytime you were nervous, your father yelled at you to "be a man?" Through conditioning, you would learn that these emotions were not good and you would most likely learn to push them deep inside.

Dealing with emotions is important for anyone. I have found in my nursing practice that many people do not deal with them in a healthy manner. I have a friend named Nita. Nita is very interested in the concepts of Buddhism. She taught me a long time ago some concepts about emotions and reality. She taught me that when I felt anxious, I should look at my feet and know that I am safe in that moment. This has helped me every time I feel myself becoming nervous about something.

As people recover and change, they learn that emotions are **not good or bad**, in themselves. **They just are.** They are a natural reaction to the reality that we think we are in. As an addiction recovery nurse, we *also learn that reality is a perception and it can be changed. We learn that we cannot change the people that are around us, but we can change the way that we react, and we can change the way that we see the situation. It is sometimes necessary to remove ourselves from the situation, so that we are able to gain this more perceptive view.*

Try this for a few seconds:

Look at your feet right now. Take a breath in your nose and breathe out of your mouth. Know that you are okay right now in this minute. Breathe in calmness and breathe out the anxiety.

Recovery is about learning to live life on life's terms. It is about adaptation, trust, and love. **You cannot give someone recovery, they have to want it.** They have to see that the pain of using is more intense than the pain of recovering. Recovery hurts. Please don't think that it doesn't. When people recover, their brains are going through changes, their bodies are going through changes, relationships are changing, and their view of the world changes as well. The pains that are felt are bitter-sweet and eventually open the recovering addict up to a whole new serene existence.

> Nothing lasts forever. Uncomfortable feelings do not last forever. They will pass if we let them. We must need to let them go. Do not hold on to them. Acknowledge them and allow them to pass. This is one of the great truths of life.

Withdrawal

My body did not always crave caffeine. I conditioned it. Quitting meant that I needed to withdrawal. I had to experience the headache and the other symptoms that presented themselves. In order to quit, I also had to be able to see that there was a true benefit to quitting. I had to believe that the pain of stopping was better than the consequences of continuing to consume caffeine. When that happened, then I was able to begin to take the first steps to change my behavior.

Quitting any habit is not easy. Anyone can agree to that. Many of our habits, we actually like. I mean, they are not getting in our way of living life. In fact, many of them make life more enjoyable – at least at first. As we change, we see that maybe all of our habits are not very good for us. We begin to think about a plan to change. We may try to summon our self-control to make this change. At first, we start off strong, but then something happens and we find ourselves back at the start line. Perhaps it was **our plan** that was faulty, maybe it was our self-will. We just need to regroup and try again.

This sequence may happen over and over again until we find the right combination. In fact, it takes many people multiple tries to change a habit. As we are changing, we just hope that the cost of partaking in the habit will not do permanent damage before we can change. This is how we grow as humans. This is how we recover from our actions of the past. So when we discuss the concept of recovery, we can substitute that word with **stopping and healing**.

Q: Can you name a habit that you consider bad that you have changed in the past? Why did you change?

Can you name something that you do that you want to change? Why do you want to change this?

Starting to Heal

Statistics say that many addicts need to try quitting a few times before they are actually able to. This is scary, because once a person is in the mist of addiction, the only places that are in his/her future is the psychiatric hospital, jail, dead, or recovering. That is where drug addictions take the user/abuser. It is the scary reality.

When you are caring for a sobering addict/abuser that they are just beginning the healing process. The earlier they are in the process, the cloudier they will most likely be. This is not the time for them to make giant life decisions. Many of the decisions that they have made to this point may have probably not been really awesome ones. Practice patience. I have not known many people who were under the influence and were making really great decisions. Usually the decisions that are made while drunk or high, are not wise at all. Think about it. When people are under the influence, their brains are firing at half-mast. This means, that if they are lucky, they are using half of their neurons and they are not working at their best anyway. When people first get sober, they think that they know what is going on, but their views are a little messed up. As the person begins to sober up, this is when the nurse must learn the language of recovery. Even if the person is not ready to recover, it is possible to plant a seed that may be grown at a future time.

Many people who have had to afford the extreme costs of addiction have had to find creative ways to finance their habit. Sometimes, they have actually learned to believe the lies that they had to tell themselves. As a nurse, please watch for this manipulative behavior. Addicts often do not mean to bring it forward, but it has been a part of their composition for so long, that they sometimes do not even realize that it is present.

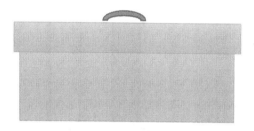

What is in Your Tool Box?

In recovery, people learn about "tool boxes." These are not a physical tool box. It is more lessons that the recovering person needs to learn and remember in recovery. Lessons like turning life's situations over to God (or a Higher Power), live and let others live the way that they choose to, what other people think about us is really not our concern (because what we think about ourselves matters the most), recovering people must also come to realize the importance of having a group of clean friends to hang out with and bounce ideas off of.

Think about it for one moment. If you had one day found yourself addicted to playing video games, and you decided that it was time to stop, would you hang around other gamers? Would you go hang out at the local video store? If you did, one might say that you were searching for trouble, right? It is the same for any addiction. If we are going to change the addictive cycle, then we need to find new places and new people to be around if we are to have a chance at recovery.

All 12-step recovery programs stress that the recovering person find a **sponsor** and a **home group**. What are these things? A home group is a recovery meeting that the person commits to go to each week. It is a group where the recovering addict knows people and the people know him/her. When he/she is not there, the members may call to see what is going on. Although any member can volunteer to help out at any meeting, the home group holds a special place in the recovering addict's heart. It is a matter of accountability.

No one can practice a 12-step program alone. It would be so overwhelming. This is why every recovering addict, finds a sponsor. A sponsor is a person in the program that often has more time than the recovering person, but more importantly it is a person that has qualities that the recovering person wants in his/her life. It is a person that the addict works through the 12 steps with. The 12-steps are the pathway to serenity and recovery. A sponsor is the person that the recovering addict calls when having a good day or a bad day. It is a person that the recovering addict can bounce ideas off of. The sponsor is a friend, but is more of a guide.

Recovering addicts can have many sponsors during their lifetime. I have heard of people having more than one sponsor at a time, although I would caution against this. It is too easy to play one against the other in this situation. If one sponsor does not say what you want them to say, then it is too easy to go to the other. The sponsor-sponsee relationship is important as many *addicts lack people in their lives that they truly trust.* As they recover, they are learning to trust again. The sponsor is usually one of the first people that the recovering addict begins to trust and love in a special way. It is therefore important for the women to have women sponsors and the men to have male sponsors. Recovering addicts do not need any more confusion in their lives. They also need to learn to trust members of our same sex. It is all about the healing.

Who do you talk to and trust when you need to talk?

How has this person/people showed you that they can be trusted?

_____

_____

_____

One of my favorite sayings is, *"but for the grace of God go I."* In other words, do not judge your fellow humans. It is by God's grace that you are not in the same situation.

Have you ever been driving down the highway and saw someone driving an old car? You may think to yourself, "Pleasssse," as you smile and acknowledge your pretty car. Is this behavior human nature? Maybe it is, but recovering addicts cannot afford this thinking. I remember back to my younger days. I bought this car that looked nice on the outside. It was a really cool color and I felt cool in it. The problem was, is that when it would start, white smoke would pour out of the exhaust. One time there were teenagers behind my car and I was about to start it. I asked them nicely to move, because I did not want them to get smoked out. They looked at me like I had three heads and said that they were fine. "Okay," I thought, "I hope you are ready." When I started my car, they started to cough and wave the smoke away. All I could think of was, "I told you so."

This story is important for a few reasons. First, if I honestly think back, I was once a teenager who thought that she knew everything. So even though I may think that they were odd, I need to remember that that was once me. In fact, if I get really honest, I still act like that from time to time. I can't tell you how many times someone has tried to show me an easier, softer way to do something, but I was determined that I was going to accomplish the task my own way. The story is also important because as I judge that person with the older car driving down the road, I had forgotten that that was once me and could easily be me again. It is, "but for the grace of God go I." The third lesson that I learned from that car is that just because something looks great on the outside, does not mean that it is great on the inside. Many things in life are wrapped in pretty packages, but they are ugly inside. This car taught me to look under the hood before I judge anything. The forth idea that I eventually learned, and this car proved, is that I do not make sound decisions sometimes. It is always a good idea to bring someone with me that knows more about the situation than I do. In other words, if I am going to buy another car, I need to bring one of my mechanic friends with me.

Another important concept in recovery is that of **gratitude.** Many people go through life wishing they had things and envying others. I think that we can all agree that this way of thinking is part of the landscaping on the serenity path. Wanting what others has is not a way to achieve happiness. When we are able to recognize and be grateful for the blessings that we have in our lives, anyone can have a chance at being content and happy. My car helped to teach me gratitude. When it started, I was happy and grateful, Unfortunately, most days it did not start, so then I became grateful that I could trade it in (even if it had to be towed into the dealership). Then I was grateful that the car dealer was able to take it off my hands. I then became grateful that I could drive home with another car that day. Then I became grateful that this newer car started when I turned the key.

Instead of having all of that gratitude, I could have chose to be mad and feel cheated about the whole thing. I could have been angry at the person who sold me that car (even though I was the one who bought it), I could have been mad at the car, I could have griped about having to pay the tow truck driver… Do you see the difference in attitudes?

Nurses are healers and when we talk to any patients, therapeutic communication is a must. This is further true when we are talking the recovery talk with patients. Watch what you say and how you say it. Learn the concept of gratitude.

Through my life, I learned to be grateful for whatever I have. Through my church, I realize that I am blessed no matter what I have. My Mom has helped me learn that stuff is just stuff. It is more stuff to dust and move around. It is not important. I went through a phase where having stuff made me happy, at least for a minute. After that minute, I became tired of the thing that I had bought. It was an awesome realization when I noted that I do not need any more stuff. In fact, I need to get rid of stuff. These are all lessons that I share when I talk recovery.

Answer this question: What makes you happy?

> *As I approach my 50's, what makes me happy is being serene. I need time alone, time with God, time with my family, and time with friends. When I am balanced in my life, I find that I am more content. I enjoy the palm trees and the warm beach. That is too bad for me though. I current live in the state of Kansas, which is smack dab right in the middle of the United States. I am as far away from any beach there is. I have learned though that I need to teach myself to be happy no matter where I am. I have learned the concept of gratitude along the way.*

Learning about the language of recovery is not reserved for recovering addicts. In fact, I have noticed that most of the concepts have come from the Bible and from famous philosophers. Recovery is about finding a spiritual pathway. It is about learning to make healthy choices. It is about living without using.

> I think that nurses, in general, are close to God. We are blessed. We get to see babies take their first breaths, and people take their last breaths. We help people heal, and we sit with them as they cross over. We see miracles every day. How could we not believe in some higher being? How could we deny ourselves this love? Nursing is love. It is about selfless caring for another. It is a profession that by its very nature is close to God.

I have seen the power of creating a gratitude list every day. **It is important to know that we are blessed even when we feel like we are not.** When we are grateful, and take care of the things that God has given us, (including ourselves) then we are at peace. It is often at this time, that I find that God gives me more. I am not talking about giving me more in stuff necessarily, God may give me more gratitude. That is a huge gift.

Please take a minute to practice the act of gratitude. It is not only a concept that religion teaches us, but if we are to pass it on to our patients who choose to recover, it must begin to be in our healing practice as well.

Today, I am grateful for:

1. _____

   _____

2. _____

   _____

3. _____

   _____

4. _____

   _____

5. _____

   _____

6. _____

   _____

7. _____

   _____

8. _____

   _____

9. _____

   _____

10. _____

   _____

If making a gratitude list is hard for you, start easy. Maybe start with, "I am grateful that I have hair (or that I don't have hair), etc."

The gratitude list should be done daily. We see that we really are able to see our life from a different point of view. We are able to be grateful for all of the things that we do have, instead of thinking about all of the things that we don't have.

> Many addicts have lost their families and friends due to their abuse. When they finally sober up, they may be in a rush to get these people back into their lives. This is normal, but it may take a lot of time. It is important to remind them again that their main priority is recovery.

As you can see, the process of recovery is complex and multi-layered. In recovery, it is important to remember, **"first things first,"** and **not to put the cart before the horse.** Recovering addicts realize that we all need to take care of the important things and then work on the rest. Sometimes, we see if we take care of the important things, the other things almost take care of themselves. It is one of the mysteries of recovery.

What is an important thing that you need to take care of today? What is your, "First thing First?"

Meditation is an important part of recovery and prayer. When I taught religious school, we were taught that prayer is talking to God and meditation is listening. Learning to take time alone with your Higher Power is vital. Some people read scripture, some sit quietly and listen, some read from a daily meditation book, while others journal. There is no right thing, as long as we are working on that relationship that we have with God.

Other books and prayers that are important to many people's recovery is the Big Book of AA, the Serenity Prayer, and the Lord's Prayer. Sobriety becomes a part of the recovering person, if he/she lets it. It begins to affect every aspect of our lives and recovering addicts then begin to receive the blessings of living a clean life. A life where God is relied upon and trust in others begins to happen. Recovering addicts learn to laugh and say that, **"our best thoughts got us where we were."** Somehow, by the grace of God, some people are able to gain sobriety. It is never taken for granted. In fact, it is often at the top of the gratitude list each day and the first part of the morning prayer. Recovering addicts know that they must always work on their relationship with their Higher Power and make prayed-upon choices. No more slippery people and places, instead they have new people in their lives, new, clean places to be, and spiritual things. They are clean and grateful. They learn to freely give away these gifts that have been given to them and they do not judge the addict that has not reached recovery. They learn to accept them, but not their disease. .

These are the basic concepts and vocabulary that should be understood by the nurse who is helping patients to recover. These concepts will be used. It is important for the addiction recovery nurse to embrace these concepts and intertwine them into his/her practice.

The Battle

Addiction is no longer a battle between "them and us," as drugs are in every society. Many people have no idea how common drugs like heroin and methamphetamines are. If you think that this is a problem that someone else deals with, you need to think again.

When I enrolled my son into high school, the school warned us that heroin was near and taught all of the parents about the signs of use/abuse. Please understand that I live in a very nice upper middle class county. These drugs are everywhere.

A Time for you to Research

What are the 12 steps?

1.

2.

3.

4.

5.

6.

7.

8.

9.

10.

11.

12.

What are the Promises of AA?

What do the promises mean and why are they important?

Part Three
Flirting with Danger

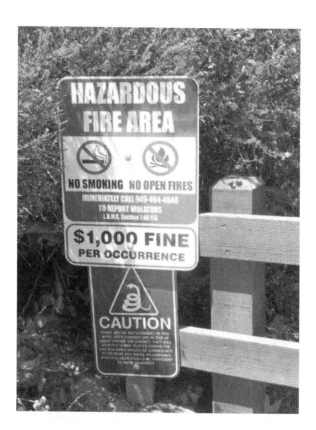

Basic Information:
Some of the Drugs of Addiction

Heroin and Other Opioids

Methamphetamine

Cocaine

Phencyclidine

K2

LSD

Marijuana

Alcohol

Ecstasy

Chapter Seven
Heroin and Other Opioids

Opioid addiction has reached a new high. It is estimated that within the United States 2.1 million people abuse prescription opioid pain killers and another 467,000 report being addicted to heroin (Theilking, 2016). Let's be real though. The only way that we know if a person is addicted to these substances is if they self-report addiction or abuse. How many people use these over-use these substances and don't say so? It is therefore my stance that these numbers are very low. Do you agree?

Who is to Blame?

Prescription pain medications abuse is high, although it is unclear how high. Everyone is looking to blame someone else. Who is to blame? There are many professionals involved in the chain of use/abuse. Where do you think that the blame should be?

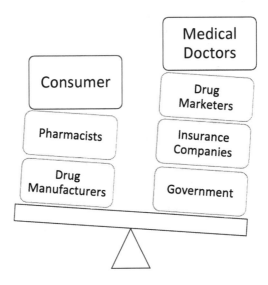

How many people think that if a medication is ordered by their doctor, that it is safe? For some reason, this seems to be a common misconception for many people. As healthcare professionals, do we review the addictive information with our patients before we administer any opioid? For years I didn't. Perhaps I was concentrating on the tasks that I needed to complete, or I thought that the patient really did not want to know anyway. Maybe I thought that they did know.

What Should We Do?

It is estimated that every year 20,000 people die from opioid overdose in America alone (Tedeschi, 2016). Based on that figure, that means that every day over 56 people die from opioid overdose. It is also known that many medical professionals in the United States have never been trained to deal with addiction (Tedeschi, 2016). So this leaves us all in a shady situation.

Opioids were and are given so freely, that in my opinion, the medical profession has created problems. Many healthcare agencies realize this issue and are taking steps to reduce the use of opioids in healthcare. In 2016, the CDC announced new guidelines for opioid prescribing (Bulloch, 2016). These guidelines are mere suggestions to medical doctors, however it is a start. In October 2016 the Drug Enforcement Agency (DEA) announced that the amount of opioids manufactured in the United States will be reduced in 2017 (Barrett, 2017). Of course, these are just two examples of agencies taking action.

Did you know that heroin is just an opioid? It has been around for years and is used in some countries like the United States uses morphine. At one point is was legal in the United States, but then our government realized that it was a little too addicting. This is when it became illegal, however if you think that it is not in circulation, think again.

If a person is addicted to pain pills and they are unable to get them, heroin is a quick substitute. The problem with many of these street drugs, is since they are not regulated by any government entity in regard to their manufacturing, it is impossible to know what is in them. Some have been cut (diluted) with hazardous materials that make the person high, but is also very dangerous to anyone's health. Many addicts say that it is so important that they know their dealer and trust them.

Why do dealers cut the drugs?

To make more money.

Opioids can be orally ingested, snorted, injected, or used in a transdermal manner. Of course, when they are injected, this is the best high, however it is the first time that is the best. Many addicts have noted that they "chase that first high." That means that they try to recreate the pure high that they had the first time that they used, however this can never be replicated. The injected high is a pure high that takes minutes to feel.

Snorting opioids is another choice for some users. Although this high is not as pure as the injected method, our nasal membranes are so vascular, that the drug is absorbed quickly. When people take these medications orally, the results can be felt in about 30 minutes. Because of the digestive system, the full effects of the drug are not felt when taken orally.

The problem with all opioids is that users build up a tolerance. In the beginning, one pill is enough, however as time continues, the user needs more and more of the medication to achieve even a moderate high. This sets a terrible, downward spiral into motion. A spiral that is scary and terrible for many people.

Opioids often give the user a mellow high. They are known as a central nervous system depressant, and should be used to treat <u>acute pain</u>. Opioids increase the amount of dopamine in our synapses. As the amount increases, many receptors shrivel away, because they realize they are not needed. Perhaps it is the body's way of protecting itself. This is how the tolerance builds. In order to feel moderate pleasure, the addict needs to increase the amount of dopamine at each receptor. For many users, that means that they need to continue using in order to avoid the physical and mental withdrawals. Physical withdrawals include nausea/vomiting, cold sweats, insomnia, yawning, fever, severe pain, involuntary kicking, anxiety, irritability, runny nose, and an intense craving to use. Many users have poor dental hygiene as a result of neglect. Physiological changes that occur while using include constipation, itching, cold sweats, sexual problems, respiratory illnesses, HIV and Hepatitis C (if used intravenously).

Two of the opioids are manufactured right from the opium poppy. These are morphine and codeine. Scientists take the plant and alter the composition to create heroin, hydromorphone, oxycodone, and hydrocodone. The lab created opioids are methadone, fentanyl, propoxyphene, meperidine and buprenorphine (Rundio & Lorman, 2015). In general, the opioids act on the mu-opioid receptor to create a sense of euphoria, relaxation and sedation (Rundio & Lorman, 2015). If a person has too much, respiratory distress often occurs.

What is the reversal drug of choice for opioid overdose?

_____

How is this drug administered?

_____

_____

_____

What does the nurse need to watch for when administering
this drug? _____

_____

_____

     The withdrawal symptoms seem to be the same for all opioids. Of course this depends on the length of time that the drug has been taken, and the amount used. Withdrawal is also known to be physically and mentally painful. This adds additional challenges for the person wishing to quit.

     Nurses are usually well versed with many of the medications that are used in the hospitals, so I will not address many of these drugs. I decided to offer some information on some of the drugs. I hope you find it useful.

Heroin

A Little More Information

Before I started to learn about many of these drugs, I really thought that many of them were a problem of modern times and were far away from my neighborhood. The more I learn, the more I see. At one point, it was legal and used in medical practice. Now it is used mostly on the streets and manufactured in make-shift labs. Heroin is an opioid, just like morphine or oxycodone. Heroin was originally made to help people recover from morphine addictions. Do you find this interesting? I do.

Heroin starts as a white of brown powder, but can also be a black sticky substance (National Institute on Drug Abuse, 2014). Heroin can be injected, inhaled, snorted, or smoked (NIDA, 2014). All of these methods cause a fast reaction in the brain.

When heroin crosses the blood brain barrier, it is converted into morphine, and then binds to the mu-opioid receptors. These receptors are located all over the brain. As a nurse, it is important to note that some of the mu-opioid receptors are located in the brain stem (NIDA, 2014). This means that blood pressure and respiration can be effected.

Chronic users can have many health problems. As they recover, it is important for the person to be evaluated by a health professional. Some of the health risks involve pneumonia, liver or kidney disease, and heart issues (NIDA, 2012). Constipation problems as well as other GI problems may also be present (NIDA, 2012).

What heart issues do you think people who are recovering from heroin may need to be screened for?

_____

_____

_____

_____

Why do you think that heroin addicts are at higher risk for a thrombus or embolus?

_____

_____

_____

_____

What medications are used to help a person withdrawal from the effects of heroin in the clinical setting?

_____

_____

_____

> When a drug is used on a regular basis, the body begins to become accustomed to having the drug present and makes adjustments as needed. When the drug is taken away, the body actually craves the drug. This is known as physical dependence.

Carfentanil

In September 2016, the DEA issued a nationwide warning pertaining to the increased use of Carfentanil (National Institute on Drug Abuse, 2016). Carfentanil is an opioid that is used to sedate large animals, such as elephants (National Institute on Drug Abuse, 2016). This drug is 10,000 times the potency of morphine, and 100 times the potency of fentanyl (National Institute on Drug

Abuse, 2016). This drug has been linked to many human deaths (National Institute on Drug Abuse, 2016). Authorities note that this drug is being added to heroin and other street drugs (National Institute on Drug Abuse, 2016).

> *As we discuss street drugs, many problems are identified. Because these drugs are not regulated and are often made in unclean labs, it is unclear what is actual ingredients are used in the creation. Users also do not know what the drug is cut with. These are many of the reasons that it is very difficult to separate the drugs into categories. More potent street drugs may also be substituted for less potent drugs. This is often a recipe for disaster.*
>
> *Post-mortem testing may not be able to identify many of these substances, so it is possible that many people will die before the substance can be identified* (National Institute on Drug Abuse, 2016).

Fentanyl

Fentanyl is a synthetic opioid that is 50 to 100 times more potent than morphine, and 30 to 50 times more potent than heroin (NIH, 2016). On the street, fentanyl is sometimes sold by itself, but more often used to lace heroin (NIH, 2016). Common street names for this drug are China Girl, China White, Goodfella, TNT, Tango and Cash, and Jackpot (NIH, 2016). When fentanyl is sold on the streets, it can be found in many forms including tablets, powder, and placed on blotter paper (NIH, 2016).

In August 2016, The Centers for Disease Control and Prevention (CDC) warning all health-care professionals about the increase in fentanyl related overdoses and deaths across the United States (NIH, 2016). Drugs that are laced with fentanyl are being sold as other opioids that are less potent (NIH, 2016). This is causing fatal overdoses to occur (NIH, 2016). The Drug Enforcement Administration has discovered that some of these pills are manufactured in China and entering the United States through the Mexican Cartels (NIH, 2016).

Desomorphine
(Krokodil)

The drug started in Russia in 2002. It has since moved to other areas of the world including the United States. This drug is highly addictive, and causes disfigurement of the user. The drug starts with codeine, however through a process, the product is cooked with toxic chemicals such as paint thinner, gasoline, and hydrochloric acid (Narconon International, 2016).

The drug was first manufactured as a remedy for those heroin addicts that could no longer afford heroin (Narconon International, 2016). However this drug is so dangerous that the average life expectancy of a user is one to two years (Narconon International, 2016). Withdrawal from this drug can cause a month or more of horrible pain (Narconon International, 2016). Very strong tranquilizers are used to combat the pain (Narconon International, 2016). If a person is able to withdrawal from the drug, permanent damage may already be present. This drug is known to cause necrosis of the muscles and cause speech impediments (Narconon International, 2016).

Did you know that there is an Opioid Withdrawal Scoring Scale that can assist healthcare professionals to help those patients withdrawal? One of the signs is yawning. What are the other signs of opioid withdrawal?

It is important to place the drugs in some order of potency. Medical professionals call this type of conversion chart an equainalgesic chart for opioids (Pharmacists Letter, 2012). When opioids are ranked, they are often compared to morphine. Please understand this is an approximation.

Drug	Strength (to oral Morphine)
Carfentanil	10,000 x
Fentanyl	50-100 x
Buprenorphine	40 x
Oxymorphone	7 x
Hydromorphone	5 x
Diamorphine (Heroin)	4-5 x
Methadone	3-4 x
Morphine IV	3 x
Oxycodone	1.5 x
Morphine Oral	

(Wikipedia, 2016)

Notes on Opioids

Chapter Eight

Methamphetamine

Street names: meth, crystal, Tina, glass, ice, crank

Methamphetamine was originally created in 1887 in Germany and then developed in Japan in 1919 (Foundation for a Drug Free World, 2006-2016). There really was no use for it until war broke out. Bomber pilots would often be given this drug so that they would be able to stay awake during flight and not be afraid if their mission ended in their demise.

Methamphetamine is a powerful, addictive stimulant. Many meth addicts talk about the first time that they tried the drug. Many claim that this was the best high they ever had. Through their use, they continue to chase this high, but can never achieve it. Methamphetamine increases the amount of dopamine in the brain (NIH, 2014).

Although methamphetamine was first manufactured legally and used in bronchial inhalers and nasal decongestants (National Institute on Drug Abuse, 2013). It is similar in chemical make up to amphetamine, however more of the chemical is able to cross the blood brain barrier

(National Institute on Drug Abuse, 2013). On the street, methamphetamine is often referred to as "meth." (National Institute on Drug Abuse, 2014). Although it is often called meth, it is also known as crystal, chalk and ice because it is often sold as a crystalline powder (National Institute on Drug Abuse, 2014). Methamphetamine can be injected, snorted, smoked, or taken orally (National Institute on Drug Abuse, 2014). It increases the dopamine in the synapses, which creates a sense of euphoria. Over time, the brain changes its chemical make-up in response to the drug. This is perhaps why this drug can lead the user to a chronic state of psychosis (National Institute on Drug Abuse, 2014).

The 2012 National Survey on Drug Use and Health (NSDUH) discovered that over 12 million people in the United States have tried methamphetamine at least one time (National Institute on Drug Abuse, 2013). Use of the drug is known to cause many health problems that medical professionals need to be aware of. Common health problems that can be associated with methamphetamine use include malnutrition, cardiac issues, anxiety, STD's, and severe dental problems (National Institutes on Drug Abuse, 2013).

Meth increases the body's temperature so high that the user passes out, often causes serious itching and can cause many mental problems (Medline Plus, 2016). Many users are known as "tweakers." The serious itching causes many people to pick at their skin until scars are formed.

Drugs that increase dopamine in the brain also often act to destroy the dopamine transporters. This means that it takes more dopamine to produce even a normal pleasure sensation. Other activities that can release dopamine include sex and certain foods. When a person stops using methamphetamine, they often do not experience pleasure with these other activities. If the addict is able to continue in recovery, these transporters often repair themselves, although this takes time (National Institutes on Drug Abuse, 2013).

Notes on Methamphetamine:

Chapter Nine

Cocaine

Street names: blow, crack, coke, snow, toot, sugar

Musicians sing about it, Hollywood glamourizes it, and it was once associated with the rich. This drug is the stimulant known as cocaine. Although it was once legal and used in common items, it is now considered an illegal substance when sold on the streets. Cocaine is still occasionally used in medical practice as a topical or local anesthesia (National Institute on Drug Abuse, 2016).

Cocaine is made from the leaves of the coca plant that is native in South America. After it is processed, it is sold on the streets as a white powder. In order to make more money, many street dealers mix (cut) the drug with substances such as talcum powder, soap powder, and cornstarch which can have serious effects on the body. Cocaine is also sometimes mixed with other drugs to create a "higher-high."

Cocaine can be snorted or injected. It can also be processed and smoked (National Institute on Drug Abuse, 2016). Cocaine increases the levels of dopamine in the brain (National Institute on Drug Abuse, 2016). It prevents the dopamine from recycling in the synapses (National Institute on Drug Abuse, 2016). Users report that the effects of cocaine are euphoria, alertness, energy, however cocaine can also cause paranoia and irritability (National Institute on Drug Abuse, 2016). Behavior is also contingent on the amount used and what the substance was cut with.

Cocaine use can have multiple detrimental effects on a person's health. Cardiac wise, it constricts blood vessels, increases heart rate and increases blood pressure as it is a stimulant (National Institute on Drug Abuse, 2016). Pupils dilate, body temperature increase, and the user may experience tremors (National Institute on Drug Abuse, 2016). The user may also exhibit signs of restlessness and nausea (National Institute on Drug Abuse, 2016). The snorting of cocaine can also cause a hole to be created in the user's nasal septum because of the vasoconstrictive properties of the drug. When the drug is cut with other substances, such as baking powder, this can often increase the rate of septal destruction.

Crack is cocaine mixed with baking soda and water. When mixed, these substances create a hardened form of the drug that resembles a rock. While in this form, the drug is able to be smoked, which is said to give the user an increased high. This makes sense when we consider the area of absorption of the lungs.

Repeated use of cocaine causes an increase of dopamine in the synapses of the neurons. As the body senses this increase in dopamine, it begins to decrease the number of dopamine receptors as a self-defense mechanism. When this happens, it makes a serious impact on the individual who is using the drug. The person becomes unable to feel pleasure under normal circumstances as there is not enough dopamine getting to through. The only way that the person can increase the level of dopamine is to use again. This is one of the ways that the drug has serious addictive qualities.

Signs of withdrawal from cocaine usually includes the inability to feel pleasure (as explained above), depression, anxiety, body aches, tremors, and depression. Although the majority of symptoms will go away unless the person uses again, the ability to feel normal pleasure may never return in some former users.

The psychological urge to use cocaine may last for years. Former users remember the times that were good, and sometimes forget the damage that the use of the drug caused. In recovery, it is very important for them to remember the complete picture.

Cocaine can cause the user to suffer from pulmonary embolisms as it constricts the blood vessels and causes changes in heart rhythms. It is also noted that sniffing cocaine through rolled money causes the spread of many diseases as money is far from clean. Cocaine use/abuse can also contribute and make many mental issues progress. Anxiety, PTSD, depression and psychosis can result or become worse.

Notes on Cocaine:

Chapter Ten

Phencyclidine

(PCP, Angel Dust, Dust, Embalming Fluid, Wack, Rocket Fuel, Hog)

Angel dust was originally brought to the market in the 1950's as an anesthetic drug, but was taken off of the market in 1965 by Parke Davis because it was causing too many issues (Drugs.com. 2000-2016).These issues included dissociative hallucinations with a sense of mania. People under the influence of PCP become very sensitive to light and sound (Dees, 2014). They also are known to have psychotic episodes (Dees, 2014).

Pain impulses are not present in the person who is under the influence of angel dust. PCP is associated with super human strength, but perhaps it is the lack of a pain impulse that creates this phenomenon (Dees, 2014). PCP causes the temperature to rise in the user, which causes many people to disrobe.

PCP is usually sold as a white crystalline powder, however it can also be sold as a liquid. PCP is synthetically made and often contains many toxic substances, such as ether or potassium cyanide when it is concerted to a liquid. This liquid PCP is known as "wet," or "water" on the streets. Cigarettes or marijuana joints are usually dipped into the liquid and then smoked. When it is smoked, it often burns the user's throat because of these flammable solvents.

PCP can be injected, smoked, taken orally, snorted, used transdermally, or sprayed onto plants (Drugs.com, 2000-2016). PCP works primarily as a NMDA receptor antagonist (Rundio & Lorman, 2015), however many dealers stretch the drug by combining it with toxic chemicals like starting fluid. This adds an extra issue for the nurse as the behavior is quite unpredictable and can often be misdiagnosed. Be aware that these additives can cause abnormal reactions to the drug.

PCP increases the amount of serotonin in the brain. It also increases dopamine and norepinephrine. It is also probable that PCP interacts with opioid and nicotinic receptors (Drugs.com, 2000-2016). Because of the chemical reactions it causes in the brain, PCP is known to continue to cause brain damage even after the user has stopped using. Hallucinations can continue even when the person is no longer under the influence (MacLaren, 2016). PCP also often leads to schizophrenia in those users who are predisposed to it. Many people do not know if they are indeed predisposed, so using this drug is quite a gamble. PCP often increases the heart rate, blood pressure and respiratory rate (MacLaren, 2016). It is known by many people on the street as the motivator of evil.

The amount that people use at one time also has an influence on the behavior that may be displayed. Doses over 5mg often are more unpredictable and the user usually feels impending doom which can lead to even more erratic behavior.

PCP, like many illegal drugs, is scary. The combination of hallucinations and no pain sensation can lead to panic, terror, and danger. Many people under the influence of this drug need to be placed in double handcuffs. If you encounter an active user in the hospital environment, use extreme caution.

> Anger management classes are very useful to recovering addicts. Many of these people have never learned how to manage their anger.

The effects of the drug can last as few as 4 hours or as long as 48 hours (MacLaren, 2016). Many times the user will feel a false sense of being invincible and may feel like their body is not their own (MacLaren, 2016).

When you hear about the man who was certain that his hand would grow back after he placed it on the train tracks, PCP may be involved. When you hear about the man who is in a panic because he sees fire coming from the center of the earth, PCP may likely be involved. When you hear about signs melting, and cars coming to life, consider PCP. Flashbacks are common with this drug, and many users continue to experience anxiety and even paranoia (MacLaren, 2016).

My Notes on PCP:

Chapter Eleven

K2

The Ever Changing Compound

A group of synthetic marijuana compounds, commonly known as "K2" have re-emerged, at least on the streets of New York (Rosenberg & Schweber, 2016). Residents often describe the users of this drug as "zombies" because of their catatonic-like behavior (Rosenberg & Schweber, 2016).

The truth is once this drug is smoked or ingested, the effects vary as the drug itself varies. If the person is predisposed to psychotic tendencies, then it is quite possible that the person may begin to show this behavior. It is therefore important for all nurses to know what these chemicals are, what they do, and the medical treatment associated with these drugs.

In recent years, scientists have discovered a set of receptors that are located in the brain and the body. These receptors are part of the endocannabinoid system (Scholastic, Inc., 2016). These endocannabinoid receptors have been found to have effects on memory, appetite, inflammation, and analgesia (Cayman Chemicals, 2016).

K2 is an umbrella name for a list of different compounds. Two compounds HU-210 and HU211 were first synthesized in 1988 at Hebrew University in Israel (NML, 2011). They were both found to have an anti-inflammatory and anesthetic properties (NML, 2011). HU-210 has been found to work by inducing special memory deficits and suppressing neurological firing in the hippocampus (Tocris, 2016). HU-211, Dexanobinol, is a central cannabinoid (CB1) and peripheral cannabinoid (CB2) agonist that has multiple effects (Cayman Chemicals, 2016). Other versions of K12 (CP 47, 497 and 497 C8) were developed by Pfizer in 1979 and 1980 for their analgesic properties (NLM, 2011). So how did all of this get out of control and into the hands of the public?

It's Marketed as What?

In retail establishments, K2 is often marketed and packaged as incense. It is found under many different names. Perhaps this is because there are so many variations of the chemical compound. It can be sold at head shops, tobacco stores, retail outlets, convenience stores, or online (DEA, 2016). Some of the common names for these chemicals have been Spice, Black Mamba, Genie Bliss, Fake Weed, Zohai and Bombay Blue (DEA, n.d.). Although the list continues to grow as the chemicals change, K2 often comes in shiny silver packages and can often look like poypourri (DEA, n.d.). K2 is often smoked through a pipe of a joint, but can also be consumed as a tea (DEA, n.d.).

K2 is often made for the streets by crushing up a herb or a plant and then spraying the substance on the leaves (NLM, 2016). Consumers never know what plants have been used and/or how much of the chemical is being used. This can cause unpredictable responses that are often very negative in nature.

Notes on K2

Chapter Twelve

Lysergic acid diethylamide (LSD)

(Acid, Microdots, Window Panes, Blotters, Loony Toons, etc.)

In 1938 Albert Hoffman was working for a pharmaceutical company, Sandoz, when he discovered LSD-25 by accident (National Geographic, 2015). He was originally working trying to create a stimulant that could aid in the respiratory system (National Geographic, 2015). When he was working with the substance one day, a small amount fell onto his skin and he began to experience the psychedelic effects (National Geographic, 2015). The Swiss pharmaceutical company produced the chemical under the name Delysic (National Geographic, 2015). By the 1965 over 40,000 patients had been given this chemical as scientists researched its use in psychiatric illnesses (Nique, 2014).

Timothy Leary (1920-1996), a psychologist, increased the popularity of this drug in the 1960's. Timothy

Leary was a college professor and researcher who advocated for the use of psychedelic drugs (BIO, 2016). He was discharged by the university when it was discovered that he and his colleagues were giving the drug to students, colleagues and inmates in an effort to study its effects (BIO, 2016). The effects were tested on many different illnesses. It is now illegal in the United States and is considered a class A, or Schedule I substance (National Geographic, 2015).

Users report an alteration of reality, increased colors, the opening of eyes to a new energy, deeper vision, etc. (National Geographic, 2015). Physical effects are confined to dilated pupils, rise in body temperature and a rise in heart rate/blood pressure (National Geographic, 2015). The more serious effects occur in the mind. LSD can make mental issues worse and bring out mental issues in those susceptible to them (National Geographic, 2015).

The effects of the drug can last as long as 12 hours and once ingested, cannot be stopped (National Geographic, 2015). Users call the feelings brought on by this drug, a "trip," (National Geographic, 2015). It is thought to work on the Serotonin type 2A receptor which is located in the frontal cortex of the brain (National

Geographic, 2015). This chemical is able to fit right into the serotonin receptors and disturb the connections (National Geographic, 2015).

The Hannover School in Germany launched a research trial to see if a non-psychodelic LSD can actually be used to treat cluster headaches (National Geographic, 2015). In the 6 patients that were tested, 5 patients reported that the cluster headaches had stopped (National Geographic, 2015). Will these studies get approval from the governments to continue?

On the streets, liquid LSD is placed on blotter paper, in gel caps, or on other substances (Nique, 2014). It is a colorless, odorless substance that can have a bitter taste when consumed (Nique, 2014).

Long term effects of this drug are still being studied. Some of the reported long term effects include flashbacks, schizophrenia, depression, anxiety, rapidly changing feelings and distorted perception of time (Nique, 2014). Since trips can be positive or negative in nature, the real threat also occurs during the trip itself. When having a bad trip, users report having a loss of judgement (Nique, 2014) and seeing things that are frightening.

It is currently estimated that over 23 million Americans have tried this drug (National Geographic, 2015).

Psilocybin
(Magic Mushrooms, Shrooms)

These mushrooms contain one of the psychiatric tryptamines psilocybin and psilocin, baeocystin or norbaeocystin (Freeman, 2016). These psychedelic mushrooms produce a feeling that is very much like LSD, however some users describe it as a mellower trip. These mushrooms are called "magic mushrooms' on the streets because of the sensation that they produce.

They are found naturally on the earth and some ancient people used them in ceremonies. In 2003 it was estimated that 8% of United States adults over the age of 26 have tried Magic Mushrooms in their lifetime (Freeman, 2016).

Whether it is LSD or mushrooms, the effects of the drug can be very dangerous. Since it is bought illegally, users never know what dose they are getting (Hallucigens.com, 2016). The effects of the drug are both dose dependent and also vary depending on who makes it. The user never knows what kind of trip he/she will experience (Hallucigens,com, 2016).

Many users experience bad trips. A bad trip is when an uncontrollable amount of anxiety, panic, fear, confusion, or combative behavior is brought about by distorted perceptions of everyday objects (Hallucigens.com, 2016). A family dog may appear very mean with teeth baring, or intense fears of death may produce delusions that cause people to act irrationally. Suicide, homicide and self-mutilation are the most irrational behavior that can be a direct result of the hallucinations brought on by this drug.

Users can also experience long term effects of the drug. Some of these effects are depression, anxiety and flashbacks (Hallucigens.com, 2016). A flash back is when the sensation of the drug comes back even when the person is not using. One use, can create occasional flashbacks that last years.

Medical Treatment

Medical management for someone who is under the influence of acid is supportive in nature, since there are no known reversal agents. Often IV fluid will be started if it is deemed safe and necessary. One on one monitoring is often wise to keep the person safe. Trips can last quite a while, so this should also be kept under consideration.

It is unknown if LSD is addicting.

Notes on LSD/Mushrooms

Chapter Thirteen

Cannabis

(Marijuana, pot, weed, etc)

Should we talk about one of the most controversial drugs ever? I guess we need to. Before we even begin, let me answer the question of addiction. Is marijuana addicting? The answer is yes. We will get into this later.

Marijuana comes from the flower of a plant. There are numerous varieties of the plant and even more are being engineered on a daily basis. These plants are often grown in warmer climates, however can be grown in a mechanically engineered environment. Marijuana (THC) is legal for medicinal purposes in some states of the United States and is legal for recreational purposes in some states too. I am not going to name the states because as time goes on, this number will most likely increase. However this is important for the nurse to know.

Marijuana is legal medically in the following states:

Marijuana is legal recreationally in the following states:

This plant has been around for thousands of years. It is not known exactly how people first began using it. Today the crushed flowers, called 'buds,' are either smoked or placed in food. There are two main species of marijuana plants. They are *Cannabis sativa and Cannabis indica* (Cervantes, 2015). C. sativa is the shorter of the two plants, has broad leaflets and is rich in cannabinol or THC (Cervantes, 2015). C. indica is a taller plant with thinner leaflets and is known as the fiber (hemp) plant because it is rich in cannabidiol or CBD (Cervantes, 2015).

Under the law, all cannabis is considered C. sativa (Cervantes, 2015). Today there are more variations than ever before. Different varieties are marketed to produce different effects in the consumer. Common effects of consuming this plant are increased appetite, calming effect, and sometimes is inspirational (Cervantes, 2015). It is important to note that some users report a feeling of paranoia. It can also cause memory, learning and behavior problems (Medlineplus, 2016). When smoked, it can also cause breathing problems and a terrible cough (Medlineplus, 2016).

Recent information states that marijuana has addictive qualities. Just like any substance, when the user crosses the line of needed to have the substance and /or the substance is effecting his/her life, there is a problem. Recent studies identify marijuana use disorder (MUD) (National Institute on Drug Abuse, 2016). The National Institute on Drug Abuse (2016) stated that over 30% of marijuana users may indeed have a degree of this disorder, although the exact percentage is unknown.

Medical Cannabis (THC) has also been found to have many medicinal qualities (Medlineplus, 2016). It has been discovered to act on the cannabinoid receptors CB1 and CB2 in the brain (National Institute on Drug Abuse,

2015). Many medications that are being considered do not give the patient the "high" part of the drug, but offer qualities like pain control and increased appetite. It should also be noted that because these medications activate the CB1 receptor, they also can cause withdrawal, psychoactive effects and dizziness (National Institute on Drug Abuse, 2015). It is also probable that users will develop tolerance to the drug (National Institute on Drug Abuse, 2015). Variations on the molecules are being tested and may prove useful in pain relief without unwanted side effects or tolerance.

Common signs of withdrawal from marijuana are irritability, anxiety, depression, mood swings and trouble sleeping. These withdrawal symptoms are currently linked to the CB2 receptor in the brain. More research needs to be done pertaining to the effects of this drug.

Cannabis Notes

Chapter Fourteen

Alcohol

It is quite possible that alcohol is one of the most dangerous drugs around. Because it is legal, inexpensive and readily available, many people think that it is okay to use or abuse. It is however, very important to note that alcohol abuse has destroyed more lives than ever thought. Alcohol use caused an estimated 88,000 deaths each year (SAMHSA, 2015). The annual estimated cost of alcohol abuse in 1992 alone was $148 billion in the United States and the cost has increased approximately 42% in recent years (Rundio & Lorman, 2015, p 5).

In 2014 over half of all Americans age 12 (yes I said 12) and over reported being a current drinker of alcohol (SAMHSA, 2015). That means that over 139 million people ages 12 and over reported using alcohol in the United States in 2014 (SAMHSA, 2015). Of these people, only 23% identified themselves as binge drinkers and 6.2% identified themselves as heavy drinkers, however 6.4% were able to be identified as having a alcohol use disorder within the past year (SAMHSA, 2015). What was quite surprising is the 2012 Behavioral Health Survey for the United States found that over 24% of 8th graders and 64% of 12th graders had used alcohol that year (SAMHSA, 2015). Considering that in the United States it is illegal to consume alcohol before the age of 21, this is a disturbing figure. It has also been identified that men are more likely to report heavy drinking than women (9.3% compared to 3.2%) (SAMHSA, 2015), however this may also be contributed to a perceived societal image of women partaking in this action.

Alcohol is absorbed through the stomach, small intestines and colon. Having food in the stomach slows the absorption process. The substance is rapidly absorbed throughout the body systems and effects almost every system. It is known to cause heart problems like arrhythmias, cardiomyopathy, high blood pressure, increased pulse rate and strokes (National Institute on Alcohol Abuse and Alcoholism, n.d.). Alcohol consumption also changes the chemical make-up of the brain and changes the way the brain looks (National Institute on Alcohol Abuse and Alcoholism, n.d.). It causes interference in the brains communication pathways which effects memory and cognition (National Institute on Alcohol Abuse and Alcoholism, n.d.).

Alcohol can also effect the liver. It can cause problems such as cirrhosis, fibrosis, alcohol hepatitis, and steatosis (National Institute on Alcohol Abuse and Alcoholism, n.d.). This is because 95% of all ingested alcohol is eliminated by the liver. It can also cause pancreatitis, and it decreases the strength of the immune system (National Institute on Alcohol Abuse and Alcoholism, n.d.). Alcohol has also shown to increase the risk of many different types of cancer (National Institute on Alcohol Abuse and Alcoholism, n.d.). Alcohol can also increase the blood glucose in the body, which complicates diabetes.

Alcoholism is about loss. As the brain chemicals are altered, hope begins to slip away. It is common for the active alcoholic to deny that anything is wrong for a long time. Perhaps this denial can be attributed to the many changes that brain undergoes with alcohol addiction.

Alcohol binds to the gamma aminobutyric acid (GABA) receptors in the brain. As this happens, the person often feels a decrease in inhibition, increased confidence, impaired judgement, ataxia and loss of fine motor control. In higher amounts, users may also experience incontinence, respiratory failure, seizures, coma and death (Rundio & Lorman, 2015). Caution against aspiration of emesis should also be taken. Some users of alcohol also report having blackouts. It is important to note that alcohol consumption greatly effects the neurotransmitter glutamate (National Institute on Alcohol Abuse and Alcoholism, n.d.). This is the neurotransmitter that is related to memory. As alcohol effects this neurotransmitter, this could be a potential cause for blackouts or lapses in memory (National Institute on Alcohol Abuse and Alcoholism, n.d.). It is important to note that blackouts occur because the brain cannot form memories, it is not because a person forgets what happens.

Unlike many other drugs, alcohol does not appear to increase the amount of dopamine in the brain. However, it does increase the amount of serotonin and causes the adrenal gland to release adrenaline. Alcohol also causes endorphins to be releases (National Institute on Alcohol Abuse and Alcoholism, n.d.). Alcohol has been found to increase the neurotransmitter norepinephrine which acts as a stimulant.

Because so many neurotransmitters are effected, the brain works hard to compensate for the changes in chemical composition (National Institute on Alcohol Abuse and Alcoholism, n.d.). These changes may actually be the reason why tolerance to alcohol occurs as well as why addiction is so prominent (National Institute on Alcohol Abuse and Alcoholism, n.d.). These changes are also why the withdrawal process off of alcohol is so dangerous and needs to be monitored by a skilled health professional. One thing is known, alcohol withdrawal has the capacity to kill the abuser.

Acute Withdrawal

When patients are admitted to the hospital, they are asked specific questions regarding their use of alcohol. If the person scores positive for chronic alcohol use/abuse/dependence, then the person it is advised that the person be placed on alcohol withdrawal protocol as explained by the hospital policies and procedures. The entire protocol usually involved a variety of lab work which includes liver enzymes, CBC, BMP and glucose. Depending on the medical doctor, additional labs may be added.

It is important for the nurse to note that people who are detoxing from alcohol can become violent. They are usually not violent people, however when the brain begins to withdrawal, behavior changes can occur. People who are detoxing can also become active and quite confused. Do not be afraid to administer lorazepam as ordered to your patient. The most important things is to keep your patient and the staff safe during this acute time.

Know your hospital's policy and do not be afraid to call the medical doctor for orders. Security can always be called for patients that are hard to control. As a last resort, consult your facilities restraint policy. Remember, it is important to use the least effective method possible to keep the patient safe.

> It is very important to identify alcohol use/abuse/addiction in your patients.

Common medications that are used to treat alcohol withdrawal are lorazepam, Haldol, valium, and phenytoin although hospital policies and drug availability may differ. Monitor ABG's on the patient and protect against aspiration. Because many active alcoholics deprive themselves of vitamins, it is important to replace vitamins (banana bag and orally) and electrolytes as indicated and ordered by the physician. Anti-emetics may also be ordered as needed, however if the withdrawal process is actively managed with sedatives, this medication may not be needed.

Alcohol withdrawal patients need close observation. Make sure that they are close to the nurses' station and that the door is open. Monitor them frequently. Make sure that the bed alarm is on, and that the bed is padded for safety. Sometimes, the alcohol withdrawal patient may also require a 1:1 sitter. Please advise the sitter to monitor the patient for increased confusion and violence. Safety always comes first.

Because cardiac arrhythmias may occur, these patients are often placed on telemetry and allowed to sleep. The nurse also needs to monitor vital signs closely and watch for alterations. If the temperature increases in the patient, consult a medical doctor before administering acetaminophen as the liver function may already be somewhat compromised.

Finally, I find it useful to monitor my alcohol withdrawal patients for any signs/symptoms of depression or suicide ideation. Also monitor them for signs of head trauma. If they were intoxicated when they arrived to the hospital, it is not clear if they suffered a head injury beforehand.

Before I close the alcohol section, please remember to work closely with your medical professional with these patients. DO not be afraid to treat as indicated and ordered. I have seen many nurses who become very afraid and nervous when they need to care for the alcohol withdrawal patient. Learn your hospital policies regarding these patients and care for them as you would care for anyone else. Their life may very well depend on your skills.

Methanol alcohol is also known as wood alcohol. It is very dangerous because it is very toxic to the body. When consumed, it often causes permanent psychiatric issues, metabolic acidosis and can quickly lead to death. These patients must be identified early. Recommended supportive treatment often involved sodium bicarb and ethanol alcohol, however medical treatments may vary depending on the provider.

Alcohol Withdrawal Scales

Alcohol withdrawal is often measured using the CIWA-Ar Scale in the acute care setting. This scale is similar in nature to the opiate COWS withdrawal scale, however it is indicated for alcohol. Ten signs/symptoms of alcohol withdrawal are measured and scored. The signs and symptoms that are scored include many of the most common indicators of acute alcohol withdrawal.

What are the 10 signs/symptoms measured with this scale?

1.

2.

3.

4.

5.

6.

7.

8.

9.

10.

What does a higher score mean to the nurse?

Physical alcohol withdrawal symptoms can begin to occur 2 hours after the last drink and have been known to last for several weeks. Psychological withdrawal symptoms may last for years. Education is vital for these patients.

Notes on Alcohol

Chapter Fifteen
3,4-methylendioxy-methamphetamine (MDMA)
(Ecstasy, Molly, X)

A 2006 report discovered that over 11 million people in America tried MDMA at least one time (Volkow, 2006).

MDMA is a synthetic combination drug that incorporates both the effects of hallucinogens and stimulants. Although it was originally used in Germany in the early 1900's, it was introduced in the 1970's as a supplement to psychotherapy (National Institute of Drugs, 2016). In 1985, it was deemed illegal by the DEA (National Institute of Drugs, 2016). MDMA comes in a variety of pill forms and are often found in the nightclub scene. They often cause the person to have an increased sense of warmth towards people, energy, pleasure, while also altering time and place (National Institute of Drugs, 2016).

MDMA's effects are caused by the chemical alteration of three neurotransmitters: dopamine, norepinephrine and serotonin (National Institute of Drugs, 2016). It is important to note that police labs report that many drugs are often mixed with MDMA (National

Institute of Drugs, 2016). These combinations can be quite dangerous and deadly (National Institute of Drugs, 2016). Some of the MDMA mixtures included "cocaine, ketamine, methamphetamine, bath salts, and over the counter cough medicines," (National Institute of Drugs, 2016). Although taking drugs without a doctor's approval is not a good idea, mixing drugs is even a worse idea.

It is unclear at this time of MDMA is physically addictive (National Institute of Drugs, 2016), however it may be psychologically addictive. Research does show that after MDMA use, many people report irritability, depression, anxiety, sleep problems and impulsiveness (National Institute of Drugs, 2016). After using MDMA, some users top the night off with marijuana.

The effects of the drug lasts approximately 3-6 hours (National Institute of Drugs, 2016). Many users may take a second and a third dose during the time they are out. This obviously increases the risk of overdose. MDMA can cause a serious rapid increase in body temperature which can lead to kidney failure (Volkow, 2006).

Notes on MDMA

Chapter Sixteen
End Note

Illegal drugs are more dangerous than ever before. Not only are they being combined, but they are being mixed with dangerous chemicals. The end note is that the consumer never knows exactly what he/she is getting. This makes overdose and death even more likely.

As a health professional these combinations make it very difficult to treat many patients who are high. If we do not know exactly what they took, then we can only use supportive therapy in many cases. We want to help in a larger way, but this is often impossible.

We must also keep ourselves safe when dealing with the patient that is actively under the influence of many of these drugs. Many people under the influence can become violent and confused. If we do not protect ourselves, there will be no one left to help these patients.

As nurses, it is vital that we continue to learn about the changing drug scene. It is really the only way that we will be able to help people who need our help. In the next chapter, I have included many additional resources that you can use to increase your knowledge. Learn some and then pass the knowledge on to your fellow nurses. If we are going to help this population, we need to work together and stay knowledgeable.

Lately, I have been reading information about new medications that are being developed that help with addiction. There is still a lot to learn about these medications. We must ask ourselves if we are in fact trading one addiction for another. Perhaps these medications will prove useful to our patients. I suppose only time will tell.

This book is meant to be an introduction to the world of addiction recovery nursing. There is more information available. Addiction recovery nursing has become so complex, however as I look deeper into it, it has also remained the same.

This book is not meant to treat a medical condition. It is meant as a nursing introductory reference

For more information, please contact:

(In no specific order)

Center for Substance Abuse Treatment

5600 Fishers Lane

Rockville, MD 20857

240-276-1660

Foundation for a Drug Free World

1-888-668-6378 (USA)

1-818-952-5260 (International)

http://www.drugfreeworld.org/home.html

National Institute on Alcohol Abuse and Alcoholism

https://www.niaaa.nih.gov/

National Institute on Drug Abuse

https://www.drugabuse.gov/publications/drugfacts/understanding-drug-use-addiction

Substance Abuse and Mental Health Services Administration (SAMHSA)

5600 Fishers Lane, Rockville, MD 20857

1-877-SAMHSA-7 or 1-877-726-4727

National Council on Alcoholism and Drug Dependence, Inc. (NCADD).

https://www.ncadd.org/about-addiction/faq/facts-about-drugs

Mayo Clinic

http://www.mayoclinic.org/diseases-conditions/drug-addiction/basics/definition/con-20020970

Drug Free Org

Partnership for Drug Free Kids

http://www.drugfree.org/

Alcoholics Anonymous

http://www.aa.org/

Hazelton Betty Ford Foundation

(866) 545-6439

www.hazelden**bettyford**.org

Part IV

Finding Peace:

Alternative Additions in Recovery

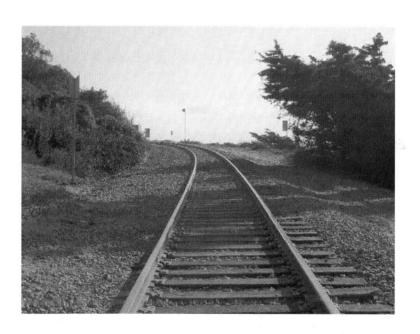

Chapter Seventeen

Why Alternative?

As a recovering addict continues the sober journey, sometimes they are reintroduced with physical and emotional pain or stress. It is important to note that there are alternative methods that can be used as part of a pain management program and as a practice that can be used to quiet the mind. A trusted medical doctor should always be consulted before trying any of these methods. This chapter is not comprehensive in any manner, but is meant to be an introduction to some of the more common alternative therapies that are available.

When Western medical practitioners discuss "alternative" methods, this traditionally means that we are discussing any method that is not considered Western.

Many times we are referring to practices that have originated thousands of years ago in China or India. Please also remember that there are many other countries and tribes that have developed their own medical practices that work well for their region. It is my belief that we must continue to learn about these methods as we consider incorporating them into the traditional medicine of many of the First World Countries.

One day I was talking to a colleague that was from Kenya. He told me of an uncle of his that was bitten by a cobra snake. The village that the family lived in was very far from any type of medical hospital and even if the family made it to the hospital, there was no guarantee that the remedy would be there. The family brought the uncle home.

In a very short time period, the uncle became very ill with fever, confusion and began to tremor. Needless to say, things were not looking very good for the uncle. All of a sudden, the grandmother came to the house with the village remedy for cobra bites. After administering to the uncle, she told the family that he would be okay. My colleague remembers seeing the uncle go from sick to well in a matter of hours. He says that he has no idea what the remedy was, but that it worked. This remedy has never been written down, but has been passed from one generation to the next. My colleague's fear is that someday this effective method may be lost.

As we discuss some alternative methods, we must keep in mind that it is vital to find a practitioner that is authentically trained in the method of treatment. It is important to talk to people and get references from practitioners if necessary. It is also important to keep an open mind.

Many comprehensive recovery houses are beginning to incorporate some of these practices into their program. The feeling is that these methods have worked for

thousands of years and warrant at least respect. So let's

take a turn and discuss some complementary therapies that

can aid and perhaps promote recovery.

Chapter Eighteen

Acupuncture

Most early civilizations did not write down their practices. Many practices from these times were passed from family member to family member through story-telling and lessons. Because of the lack of formal record keeping, it is challenging to state when acupuncture began. Today's historians are quite certain that acupuncture originated in China. There is written proof that it was used as a therapy in 100 BCE, although it is possible that it was used as early as 6000 BCE (White and Ernst, 2004). Acupuncture is a treatment that is used to prevent and treat disease (Gao, 1997).

Learning the art of acupuncture takes many years and is quite complicated. It is based on the meridians and collaterals. These meridians and collaterals create pathways in the body (Gao, 1997).The internal pathways connect to the internal organs while the exterior pathways connect to the skin (Gao, 1997). It is through all of these pathways that the energy (Qi) flows.

There are 12 regular meridians. Six of these are Yin channels and six of these are Yang channels (Gao, 1997). The six Yang channels are

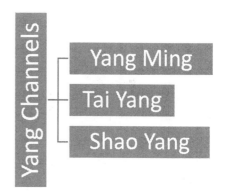

further divided into Yang Ming, Tai Yang and Shao Yang and the six Yin channels are divided

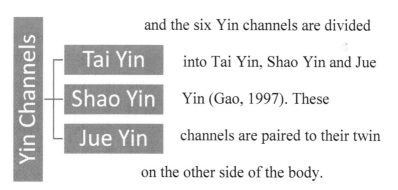

into Tai Yin, Shao Yin and Jue Yin (Gao, 1997). These channels are paired to their twin on the other side of the body.

Aside from the 12 regular meridians, there are also 8 extra meridians that are also called the extraordinary vessels (Gao, 1997). These meridians act as the reservoirs for Qi, blood and essence (Gao, 1997). What is important to remember is that these meridians and collaterals must be clear to be able to have the energy flow.

Extraordinary Vessels

- The Conception Vessel
- The Governing Vessel
- The Penetrating Vessel
- The Girdle Vessel
- The Yin and Yang regulating vessels
- The Yin and Yang motility vessels

When injury takes place in our body, the energy is not able to flow which causes further damage. It is also important to note that organs are interconnected. When one organ suffers, other organs suffer as well.

What is very interesting is that acupuncturists believe that a condition in an organ presents itself in other manners. For instance, when something is wrong with the heart, it effects the small intestines, and follows to the tongue (Gao, 1997). When the heart is sick, it shows in the face of the person (Gao, 1997). The lungs are connected to the large intestine and open to the nose (Gao, 1997). Ailments in the lungs are shown in the condition of the skin and in the body hair (Gao, 1997). The spleen is related to the stomach, opens into the mouth and controls the muscles and limbs (Gao, 1997). When the spleen is injured, we are able to see this in the person's lips (Gao, 1997). The liver is related to the gall bladder, opens to the eyes and is in charge of the ligaments (Gao, 1997). It is reflected in the condition of the nails (Gao, 1997). The kidneys are related to the bladder, open to the ears, the anus and the urethra (Gao, 1997). They are in charge of the bones and are reflected by the hair on the head (Gao, 1997).

Before acupuncture can begin, the person must be diagnosed. Chinese medicine uses four methods to evaluate a person's condition. These four methods are observation, olfaction (smelling), interrogation (asking questions) and auscultation (hearing and palpation) (Gao, 1997). It is thought that the best comprehensive picture of the person's health is brought about by using many senses. Just as medical diagnosis takes a trained professional. Diagnosis of conditions from a Chinese medical standpoint also takes a trained professional.

Observation in Chinese medicine involves noting the person's general appearance (Gao, 1997). This includes the person's "vigor, stance, color of the facial complexion, and the movements and responses of the patient," (Gao, 1997, p 189). Also included are observations of the skin, hair, nails, mouth, tongue, nose and eyes (Gao, 1997). It is important to note that the practitioner takes a lot of time during the assessment period.

Chinese medicine and acupuncture does not rely on expensive machines to diagnose, as many of these tests were not available in early times. They were not needed either. Once the blocked pathways are determined, then the practice of acupuncture can begin.

The practice of acupuncture involves inserting very thin needles into some of the 350 identified points on the body. The needles are inserted at various depths. People who have received acupuncture state that it is not painful. Many studies have been completed that tested the effects of acupuncture. All were positive. The World Health Organization (WHO) stated that acupuncture is helpful in treating at least 28 conditions (Nordqvist, 2016).

Most sessions last from 30 minutes to an hour. The total treatments required for most illnesses involve no more than 12 sessions (Nordqvist, 2016). The needles are inserted and stay in place for about 20 minutes (Nordqvist, 2016).

Acupuncture is not for everyone and it is important that the patient consult their medical doctor before starting this therapy. It is known as an alternative therapy and appears to work quite well in controlling pain. Acupuncture should not be used in most people who have a bleeding disorder or are on blood thinners (Nordqvist, 2016). It is also important that the patient make sure that the needles are sterile (Nordqvist, 2016).

Interesting fact

The United States Air Force started to teach battlefield acupuncture to physicians who were being sent to Afghanistan and Iraq in 2009 (Nordqvist, 2016).

Acupuncture is being more widely used in a variety of ways. It has become an important part of Western Medicine as an alternative for pain medication and as a healing source for many illnesses. Modern thoughts state that health professionals need to become more educated in the practice so that a better understanding can be gained.

"Open your mind to all of the

possibilities."

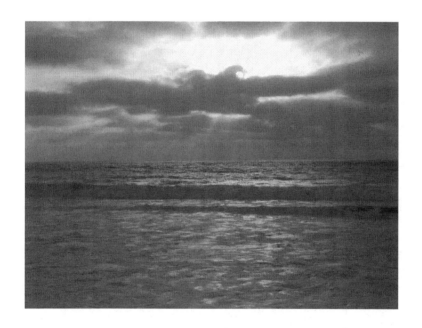

Chapter Nineteen

Tai Chi

The martial art form known as Tai Chi was said to have originated from a Taoist Priest who lived in a temple in China's Wu Dong Mountains (Standford, n.d.). One day, as the Priest was outside, he noticed a beautiful white cranes movements. As he noted the beauty of the animal's movements, he began to imitate them. As a result, the art of Tai Chi was born.

The practice of Tai Chi has been found to decrease stress, increase flexibility and decrease pain. Although it was originally developed as a form of self-defense, the slow controlled movements have been found to aid in healing and in stress reduction (Mayo Clinic Staff, 1998-2016).

Tai Chi originated in China and is also called tai chi chuan (Mayo Clinic Staff, 1998-2016). The controlled, focused movements and deep controlled breathing have great benefits. Although there are many variations of Tai Chi, each one is low impact and can be practiced by most age groups.

Tai Chi can improve balance, coordination and stability in everyone, but is especially useful in older people (National Center for Complementary and Integrative Health, 2006). It has been shown to be useful in reducing back pain, knee pain, and improving the quality of life in people who suffer from Parkinson's disease, heart disease, cancer and many other chronic illnesses (National Center for Complementary and Integrative Health, 2006).

It is best to learn Tai Chi from a person who is knowledgeable in the practice. This helps to assure that the movements are practiced correctly. After the movements are learned, tai chi can be practiced anywhere, including outside.

> *I visited Southern California recently. As I walked to one of my favorite parks, I noted an outdoor Tai Chi class. This group of people were practicing Tai Chi on a hill that overlooked the ocean. What a perfect place to practice the art of Tai Chi.*

Chinese Martial Arts

There are more than 300 martial arts styles practiced in China (Standford, n.d.). These martial art styles are divided into external and internal systems (Standford, n.d.). The external movements emphasize "linear movements, breathing combined with sound, strength, speed and hard power impact contact, jumps and kicks," (Standford, n.d.). The internal styles include Tai chi and emphasize stability with limited jumps and kicks (Standford, n.d.).

There are also many different types of Tai Chi Chuan. Of all of the types there are five that are commonly practiced: Yang, Chen, Wu, Sun and Woo (Standford, n.d.). It is important to note the type of Tai Chi that you are learning. Consulting your medical doctor is also important before starting any exercise program.

Reflection through questions: What benefits could a recovering addict find in practicing Tai Chi?

Chapter Twenty

Massage Therapy

If you have ever had a professional massage, you never forget the relaxed feeling it created.

Massage therapy involves the manipulation of soft body tissues. Massage therapy is thought to improve a person's health and well-being as they decrease stress, reduce anxiety, relax muscles, reduce pain, and rehabilitate injuries (Northwestern Health Sciences University, 2016).

Massage therapy also originated in China over 3,000 years ago (Associated Bodywork & Massage Professionals, 2016). Egyptians, Hindus and Persians also believed in the healing power of massage therapy (Associated Bodywork & Massage Professionals, 2016). Many massages include the use of scented oils that are meant to relax the person. This is called an aromatherapy massage.

There are many types of massages that a person can chose from. Each massage uses a slightly different technique. The more common massage therapies in the United States are currently:

- The Swedish Massage: characterized by long, smooth strokes and kneading on superficial layers of muscle (Wong, 2016). Often referred to as a traditional massage. It is very gentle and relaxing (Wong, 2016). The therapist can adjust the pressure used depending on the wishes of the client.

- The Hot Stone Massage: The hot stone massage incorporates heated stones that are placed on certain points of the body to warm and relax tightened muscles (Wong, 2016). The stones are often placed in a row down the spine, in the hands and on the legs. After they are placed, the stones remain in place for a few minutes and may be manipulated by the therapist. The hot stone massage is thought to aid in balancing the energy in the body (Wong, 2016).

- The Deep Tissue Massage: As the name implies, this massage works on the deeper tissue and muscles (Wong, 2016). This massage is often intense and can be slightly painful at first. "Deep tissue massage is used for chronically tight or painful muscles, repetitive strain, postural problems, or recovery from injury," (Wong, 2016). Because of the intensity of the massage, people often feel sore for a couple of days after the massage (Wong, 2016).

- Thai Massage: Using specific points on the body, this massage helps to realign the energy flow (Wong, 2016). This type of massage is very interactive. In fact, it is closely related to yoga with an instructor. It is stretching and energizing form of massage therapy. Before embarking on this type of massage, please find out more information.

Reflexology and Reiki

In this section I am going to discuss reflexology and Reiki. Although they are not traditional massage therapy, they have their place in health. It is important for the nurse to understand what they are and how they work.

Reflexology uses pressure points on the feet, hands and ears to improve specific organs and body systems (University of Minnesota, 2016). Similar to acupuncture, reflexology has identified specific points on the feet, hands and ears that are connected to the functioning of specific locations on the body. When these points are manipulated, the energy that flows is opened and the overall health of the area can be improved.

Reflexologists use maps of the feet, hands and ears to know where to manipulate. These maps are actually quite complicated. Reflexology uses "zone therapy" which identifies energy streams. Through manipulation of the outside points, the muscles relax and the blood flow through these streams is then opened up.

Reiki is a Japanese technique that helps reduce stress and can promote healing (The International Center for Reiki Training, 1990-2016). Reiki is practiced through the laying on hands and operates through the idea that there is energy field in all of us (The International Center for Reiki Training, 1990-2016). This life force field can be transferred through proper positioning and training.

The word Reiki is made up of to Japanese words. The first word is REI which translates to the Higher Power's Wisdom, and KI which refers to the energy of the life force (The International Center for Reiki Training, 1990-2016). Reiki has been shown to help in every known illness and is said to always create a beneficial effect (The International Center for Reiki Training, 1990-2016). Reiki can be practiced on yourself, but is often practiced with a trained Reiki practitioner. Reiki can even be used on animals!

Practice Reiki:

On the main page for The International Center for Reiki Training, there is a five (or so) minute video that demonstrates Reiki hand positions for self-healing. This video can be found at

http://www.reiki.org/faq/whatisreiki.html and is also available on YouTube. At this time, or as soon as possible, try these 4 Reiki healing positions. Keep an open mind and see what you think.

Chapter Twenty-One

Meditation

There are many types of meditation available, however the basic practice means quieting one's mind and relaxing. Mediation concentrates on deep breathing and being mindful of the sounds around us. Meditation allows us to slow down our world for a few minutes and center ourselves.

Over recent years, many studies involving mediation have been completed. Some of these researchers found that the practice of mediation can actually cause positive brain changes (Walton, 2015). Changes in the grey matter, enhanced connectivity, and reduced activity in the "me" centers of the brain are just a few of the measurable changes noted in these studies (Walton, 2015). Practitioners

of mediation will tell you that the practice decreases

anxiety and increases a sense of being connected with the

world. Scientists have stated that the practice of meditation

decreases depression and anxiety, improves concentration,

and improves overall psychological well-being (Walton,

2015). Meditation has also been shown to preserve the

working capacity of our brains longer (Walton, 2015).

Walton (2015) explained a study that was

conducted by researchers at Yale on meditation. These

researchers found that mindfulness meditation actually

decreased the activity in the brains default mode network

(DMN) (Walton, 2015). The DMN is the part of the brain

that has many responsibilities. Some of these

responsibilities include freethinking, remembering the past,

planning for future events and relating to others thoughts

(Buckner, Andrews-Hanna and Schacter, 2008). In 2011

Sara Lazar and her research team at Harvard, found that

meditation can actually increase cortical thickness in the hippocampus, while decreasing brain cell volume in the amygdala (Walton, 2015).

There are many ways to meditate and there are many centers that teach the art. If a person is not able to find or get to a center, there are many useful tools on-line. The nurse can be trained in guided imagery and mediation. It is then possible to work with patients with this healing technique.

Mediation has also been found to help with addiction because it effects the self-control regions of the brain (Walton, 2015). Meditation helps the person ride the craving until it passes (Walton, 2015). Meditation also allows the person to relax and think the thought through.

Active Learning:

Find a mediation on-line and try it. Quiet your mind and follow the meditation. See how you feel afterwards.

Chapter Twenty-Two

Wrapping it up

There are many other areas of holistic medicine that can be practiced with the person who is in the process of recovering. Many of the methods have been practiced for thousands of years and are not known to lead to any addiction. Combined with a recovery program, these methods can prove to be priceless. Some of these methods can be practiced alone and are not expensive at all, where others require a specially trained person to perform the technique. Always check with your medical doctor before starting any of these therapies.

We have discussed acupuncture, massage therapy, reiki, meditation, tai chi and reflexology. There are many more practices that can be incorporated into healing. Some of these practices are:

- Aromatherapy
- Nutrition therapy
- Cupping
- Imagery
- Qigong
- Yoga
- Exercise
- Tui na
- Breath work
- Sowa Rigpa (Tibetan Medicine)
- Prayer
- Acupressure
- many more

It is important for the addiction recovery nurse to be mindful and open to learning about many of these practices.

They are becoming more popular in Western Medicine. California is probably the leader in implementation. For more information on holistic nursing practices, please consult *the American Nurses Association (ANA) Scope and Standards of Practice: Holistic Nursing.*

For additional information on the various forms of holistic medicine, I have created the following list.

American Holistic Nurses Association
Certification available, education, research, resources, membership.
www.Ahna.org
2900 SW Plass Court
Topeka, KS 66611-1980
800-278-2462

International Center for Reiki Training
http://www.reiki.org/faq/whatisreiki.html
Free downloads, Reiki News Magazine, Reiki Articles, videos, free online newsletter and more.

More about healing practices?

Take a visit to the University of Minnesota, Center for Spirituality & Healing at http://www.takingcharge.csh.umn.edu/explore-healing-practices/reflexology
or
http://www.csh.umn.edu/
612-624-9459

UCLA Mindful Awareness Research Center

Online classes available.

Free Guided Meditations available online.

http://marc.ucla.edu/body.cfm?id=22

When I started this journey of recovery, I never thought that it would be so magical sometimes and so hard at other times.

`Anonymous

Chapter Twenty-Three

Healing

Recovery from addiction is about healing. This healing does not take place overnight. It in fact, seems to take a lifetime of learning about oneself. It is about learning to quiet the mind and feel the sense of connection with life. It is about learning to live life on life's terms and giving back along the way.

It seems that the only way to recover is to practice abstinence. By avoiding the first use, the recovering addict enjoys freedom from the pull of the drug. The current thought on recovery is that it needs to be holistic in nature.

It is important for the recovering person to have a plan in place for when triggers are activated. As they ask themselves what they will do when they want to use, they must have an answer as these times will surely come. Going to meetings, calling a recovery friend, helping another or reading literature all seem to be useful.

Alternative methods are meant to enhance this journey. They should not take the place of any part of the recovery practice, but these practices can all be used to compliment life. Doing positive things for oneself is an essential part of recovery. We learn to forgive and love ourselves.

I hope this book has been useful as an introduction to the world of addiction and recovery. There is much to learn. At this time, we only know a little, however a little is enough to help millions of people regain their lives.

The medical community needs to continue to talk about this epidemic and offer assistance to the suffering addict. It is through this relationship, that many people can become whole again. There are many organizations and certifications that are available to nurses who are interested in addiction recovery. Some of these are:

International Nurses Society on Addictions (IntNSA)

http://www.intnsa.org/

Certification: Certified Addictions Registered Nurse (CARN)

American Society for Pain Management Nursing

http://www.aspmn.org/certification/Pages/certification.aspx

Certification: Pain Management Nursing Certification, RN-BC

The American Holistic Nurses Association

ahna.org/

Certification: Holistic Nursing Certification

Be the change that you want to see in

the world. Give yourself to others.

Share your knowledge and most

important, be present.

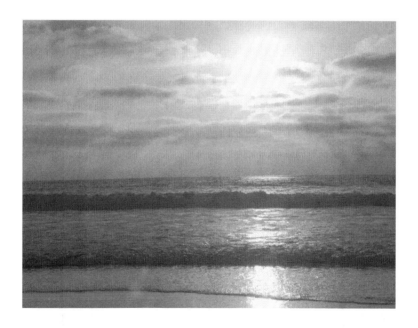

A Note about the Salvation Army

Since half of all proceeds from this book will be given to the Salvation Army Adult Recovery Center in Kansas City, MO, I decided to place a little history of the Salvation Army here. This book is not affiliated with them, but is written in honor of them.

The Salvation Army was a dream and mission of William Booth. In 1865 Booth left the standard Methodist Ministry to preach to the people that lived in the slums of London (Salvation Army, 2013). These were the people that were not very welcome in the churches at the time. Booth decided that everyone needed to hear God's word, so he opened up Christian Mission Centers in many of London's poor areas so that he could help the poor and forgotten (Salvation Army, 2013). Booth set up his church to resemble an army and established himself as the General (Salvation Army, 2013). Booth stated that his army would fight for salvation, and the name stuck. Together in their armor, the Salvation Army sought to help the homeless, poor, and the hungry (Salvation Army, 2013). In 1882 William Booth converted an old Oxford Street ice skating rink into a place of worship in 1882 (Fletcher, 2015). In his church, Booth welcomed everyone with open arms. Outside the back entrance, many homeless men would gather waiting for the drop-in center to open (Fletcher, 2015). Booth described these men as, "the least, the last and the lost," as they were often jobless and on their last chance (Fletcher, 2015).

Many of these men were drug addicts, alcoholics, physically sick, mentally ill, and some were even soldiers who suffered from PTSD (Fletcher, 2015). Booth believed that if you give a man some soap, some soup, and some salvation, that they will gain a new attitude while finding purpose (Fletcher, 2015). Today, the same mission holds true.

Booth's mission did not come without resistance from some of the people. Brothel owners and brewers were often threatened by Booth's messages (Fletcher, 2015). Mobs would often throw stones at Booth and his Army. In fact, in the early days, the women would wear specially selected bonnets to protect their heads from the stones that the crowds might throw at them.

The Salvation Army reached the United States in 1879 and by the early 1900's, the Army had thousands of soldiers and could be found in 36 countries (Salvation Army, 2013). Today the Salvation Army has thousands of centers and helps people in over 100 countries in a multitude of ways (Salvation Army, 2013).

One of the ways that the Salvation Army is able to help many people is through their many adult recovery centers, like the one in Kansas City, MO. These centers are all over the United States, and quite possibly the world. The Kansas City Salvation Army Adult Recovery Center is able to house 130 men who choose to work to recover from substance abuse. The program is free of cost to the men, but it is not easy. Their daily schedules are quite regulated between work-therapy, bible study, counseling, and meetings. The program is six months in length and involves five stages of recovery exercises.

The center is currently operated by Majors Mary and Michael, although many other people work very hard to make the center a great. The center is funded by private donations, but also from the profits of eleven of the areas retail stores. Many men have sobered up in this center over the years and many more continue to get their life changed for the better.

I am blessed to be able to not only volunteer there, but I also bring nursing students there for one of the local universities. This book was written for them, and for any other nurse who is interested in addiction recovery nursing. Thank you for your support.

Disclaimer

As a disclaimer, I am writing this book as an individual nurse. This book is in no way affiliated with the Salvation Army or any of its volunteers, employees or beneficiaries. This book is written with love as a basic education tool for nurses. It is not meant to diagnose or treat any ailment or addiction. It is meant for basic informational purposes only.

References

Alcoholics Anonymous (2001). *Alcoholics Anonymous (4ᵗʰ ed)*. New York, NY: Alcoholics Anonymous World Service, Inc.

Alcoholics Anonymous (2016). Information for professionals. Retrieved from: http://www.aa.org/pages/en_US/information-for-professionals

Alcoholics Anonymous General Service Office (2016). Estimates of AA groups and members as of January 1, 2016. Retrieved from: www.aa.org/assets/en_US/smf-53_en.pdf

Allsop, D., Norberg, M., Copeland, J., Fu, S. & Budney, A.J. (2011, December). The Cannabis Withdrawal Scale Development: Patterns and predictors of cannabis withdrawal and distress. Drug and Alcohol Dependence 119 (1-2), 123-129, doi: 10.1016/j.drugalcdep.2011.06.003

Armstrong, D. (2016). Secret trove reveals Abbot's bold 'crusade' tp sell OxyContin. Retrieved from https:www.statnews.com/2016/09/22abbott-oxycontin-crusade

Associated Bodywork & Massage Professionals (2016). Learn. Retrieved from http://www.massagetherapy.com/learnmore/

Atlantic Monthly Group (2016). A brief history of opioids:

Pain, opioids and medicinal use. Retrieved from

http://www.theatlantic.com/sponsored/purdue-
health/a-brief-history-of-opioids/184/

Barrett, J. (2016). DEA reduces opioid manufacturing for

2017. Retrieved from

http://www.pharmacytimes.com/news/dea-reduces-
opioid-manufacturing-for-
2017?utm_source=Informz&utm_medium=Pharma
cy+Times&utm_campaign=PT_Breaking_News_1
0-4-16

BIO (2016). Timothy Leary. Retrieved from

http://www.biography.com/people/timothy-leary-37330#film-tv-tech

Buckner, R., Andrews-Hanna, J., and Schacter, D. (2008).

The brains default network: Anatomy, function and

relevance to disease. Doi:10.1196/annals.1440.011

Retrieved from

http://psych.colorado.edu/~hannaje/publications_%
26_cv_files/buckner_et_al_anyas_2008.pdf

Bulloch, M. (2016). New strategies for opioid stewardship.

Retrieved from

http://www.pharmacytimes.com/contributor/marily
n-bulloch-pharmd-bcps/2016/06/new-strategies-
for-opioid-stewardship/p-2

Casey, E. (1978). History of drug use and drug users in the
United States. Retrieved from
http://www.druglibrary.org/schaffer/history/casey1.
htm

Cayman Chemicals (2016). HU-211. Retrieved from
https://www.caymanchem.com/product/100006350

Centre for Addiction and Mental Health (CAMH) (2001).
Clinical Institure Withdrawal Assessment For
Alcohol (CIWA). Retrieved from
http://www.reseaufranco.com/en/assessment_and_tr
eatment_information/assessment_tools/clinical_insti
tute_withdrawal_assessment_for_alcohol_ciwa.pdf

Cervantes, J. (2015). *The Cannabis Encyclopedia* (p 14).
China: Van Patten Publishing.

Dees, T. (2014). What is it like to do angel dust? Retrieved
From
https://www.quora.com/What-is-it-like-to-do-angel-
dust

Dossett, W. (2013). Addiction, spirituality and 12-step
programmes. *International Social Work 56*(3), 369-
383, doi:10.1177/0020872813475689.

Drug Enforcement Agency (DEA)(n.d.). Fact sheet: K2 or
 Spice. Retrieved from
 https://www.dea.gov/druginfo/frug_data_sheets/K2
 _Spice.pdf

Drugs.com (2000-2016). PCP (Phencyclidine). Retrieved
 from https://www.drugs.com/illicit/pcp.html

Encyclopedia Britannica (2016). Temperance movement.
 Retrieved from
 https://www.britannica.com/topic/temperance-
 movement

Fletcher, M. (2015). The least, the last, and the lost: As the
 Salvation Army marks its 150th anniversary, what
 role does it have to play in this secular age? *New*
 Statesman, 34-39.

Foundation for a Drug-Free World (2006-2016). Alcohol.
 Retrieved from
 http://www.drugfreeworld.org/drugfacts/alcohol/a-
 short-history.html

Foundation for a Drug-Free World (2006-2016). Retrieved
 from http://www.drugfreeworld.org/home.html

Freeman, S. (2016). How magic mushrooms work.
 Retrieved from
 http://science.howstuffworks.com/magic-
 mushroom.htm

Gao, D. (1997). *Traditional Chinese Medicine.* London, WIT: Carlton Books.

Hallucigens.com (2016). 5 dangerous LSD drug effects. Retrieved from http://hallucinogens.com/lsd-acid/5-dangerous-lsd-drug-effects/

International Center for Reiki Training (1990-2016). What is Reiki? Retrieved from http://www.reiki.org/faq/whatisreiki.html

MacLaren, E. (2016). The effects of PCP use. Retrieved from http://drugabuse.com/library/the-effects-of-pcp-use/

Mayo Clinic Staff (1998-2016). Tai chi: A gentle way to fight stress. Retrieved from http://www.mayoclinic.org/healthy-lifestyle/stress-management/in-depth/tai-chi/art-20045184

Medline Plus (2016). Marijuana. Retrieved from https://medlineplus.gov/marijuana.html

Medline Plus (2016). Methamphetamine. Retrieved from: https://medlineplus.gov/methamphetamine.html

Narconon (2016). Krokodil information. Retrieved from: http://www.narconon.org/drug-information/krokodil.html

National Drug Intelligence Center (2012). National drug
Threat assessment. Retrieved from:
https://www.justice.gov/archive/ndic/

National Geographic (2015). LSD. Retrieved from
https://www.youtube.com/watch?v=W_fqquz0Ug8

National Institute on Alcohol Abuse and Alcoholism (n.d.).
Alcohol's effect on the body.
Retrieved from https://www.niaaa.nih.gov/alcohol-
health/alcohols-effects-body

National Institute on Drug Abuse (2016, June). Drug facts:
Cocaine. Retrieved from
https://www.drugabuse.gov/publications/drugfacts/c
ocaine

National Institute on Drug Abuse (2016). Drug facts:
Fentanyl. Retrieved from
https://www.drugabuse.gov/publications/drugfacts/
fentanyl

National Institute on Drug Abuse (2014). Drug facts:
Heroin. Retrieved from
https://www.drugabuse.gov/publications/drugfacts/
heroin

National Institute on Drug Abuse (2015, April).
Cannabinoid receptor 2: Pain treatment without

tolerance or withdrawal. Retrieved from
https://www.drugabuse.gov/news-events/latest-science/cannabinoid-receptor-2-pain-treatment-without-tolerance-or-withdrawal

National Institute on Drug Abuse (2013). Research report series: Methamphetamine. Retrieved from:
https://www.drugabuse.gov/publications/research-reports/methamphetamine/letter-director

National Institute on Drug Abuse (2014). Drug facts: Methamphetamine. Retrieved from:
https://www.drugabuse.gov/publications/drugfacts/methamphetamine

National Institute on Drug Abuse (2016, October). Drug facts- MDMA (Esctasy/Molly).
Retrieved from
https://www.drugabuse.gov/publications/drugfacts/mdma-ecstasymolly

National Institute on Drug Abuse (2016). Emerging trends and alerts. Retrieved from:
https://www.drugabuse.gov/drugs-abuse/emerging -trends-alerts.

Nique, D. (2014). LSD: The trippy truth. Retrieved from
https://prezi.com/aoyv-6dqajxx/lsd-the-trippy-truth/

NML (2011). Cannabicylohexanol. Retrieved from

https://toxnet.nlm.nih.gov/cgi-
bin/sis/search/a?dbs+hsdb:@term+@DOCNO+8002

Nordqvist, C. (2016). Acupuncture: How does acupuncture
work? Retrieved from
http://www.medicalnewstoday.com/articles/156488.
php

Northwestern Health Sciences University (2016). What
is massage therapy? Retrieved from
https://www.nwhealth.edu/school-of-massage-
therapy/massage-therapy-definition/

Open Bible (2016). Drunkards. Retrieved from
https://www.openbible.info/topics/drunkards

Patterson, E. (2016). History of drug abuse. Retrieved from
http://drugabuse.com/library/history-of-drug-abuse/

Pharmacists Letter (2012). Equiamalgesic dosing of opioids
for pain management. Retrieved from
https://www.nhms.org/sites/default/files/Pdfs/Opioi
d-Comparison-Chart-Prescriber-Letter-2012.pdf

Rosenberg, E. and Schweber, N. (2016). 22 suspected of
overdosing on synthetic marijuana in Brooklyn.
New York Times. Retrieved from
http://nyti.ms/290pliH

Rundio, A. & Lorman, W. (2015). Curriculum of Addiction
Nursing (3rd ed). New York, NY, Wolters-Kluwer.

Sacred Connections (2009). The history of Alcoholics
    Anonymous: Oxford Group's influence. Retrieved
    from
    http://www.12wisdomsteps.com/related_topics/hist
    ory/oxford_movement.html

SAMHSA (2015). Alcohol. Retrieved from
    http://www.samhsa.gov/atod/alcohol

Scholastic, Inc. (2016). The science of endocannabinoid
    system: How THC effects the body and the mind.
    Retrieved fro
        http://headsup.scholastic.com/students/endo
    cannabinoid

Soong, J. (2005-2016). New to massage: FAQ: What to
    expect from your first massage. Retrieved from
    http://www.webmd.com/balance/features/massage-
    types-and-techniques

Standford (n.d.). A history of Tai Chi Chuan. Retrieved
    from
    http://web.stanford.edu/group/taichi_wushu/taichi.h
    istory.html

Substance Abuse and Mental Health Services
    Administration (2016). Center for Substance Abuse
    Treatment. Retrieved from:

http://www.samhsa.gov/about-us/who-we-
are/offices-centers/csat

Tedeschi, B. (2016. Watching the ship sink': Why primary
care doctors have stayed out of the fight against
opioids. Retrieved from
https://www.statnews.com/2016/10/19/primary-
care-doctors-opioid-treatment/

Theilking, M. (2016). John Oliver tackles the opioid crisis.
Retrieved from
http://us11.campaign-
archive2.com/?u=f8609630ae206654824f897b6&id
=40f82d1792

Tocris (2016). HU-210. Retrieved from
http://www.tocris.com/sispprod.php?Itemid=2257#
.V4eLQ_krL3Q

University of Minnesota (2016). Reflexology: What is
Reflexology? Retrieved from
http://www.takingcharge.csh.umn.edu/explore-
healing-practices/reflexology

Volkow, N. (2006). A letter from the editor. Retrieved from
https://www.drugabuse.gov/publications/research-
reports/mdma-ecstasy-abuse/letter-director

Walton, A. (2015). 7 ways meditation can actually change

the brain. Retrieved from
http://www.forbes.com/sites/alicegwalton/2015/02/
09/7-ways-meditation-can-actually-change-the-
brain/#14a07d807023

Wesson, D. and Ling, W. (2001, April-June). The clinical
opiate withdrawal scale (COWS). *Journal of
Psychoactive Drugs 35*(2). Retrieved from
https://www.researchgate.net/profile/Donald_Wesso
n2/publication/10608525_The_clinical_opiate_with
drawal_scale_COWS/links/571957a408ae30c3f9f2c
232.pdf

White, A. and Ernst, E. (2004). A brief history of
acupuncture. *Rheumatology* (43), 662-663.
Retrieved from
http://rheumatology.oxfordjournals.org/content/43/
5/662.short#

Wikipedia (2016). Opioid equivalency table. Retrieved
from https://en.wikipedia.org/wiki/Equianalgesic

Wong, C. (2016). 10 most popular types of massage.
Retrieved from
https://www.verywell.com/most-popular-types-of-
massage-89741

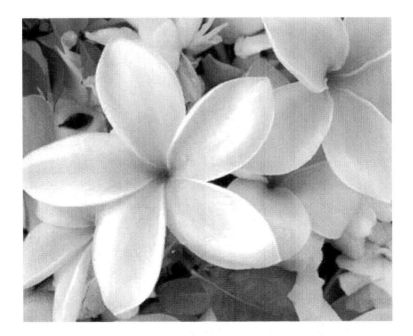

Published by:

Lauranda Publishing

Overland Park, KS

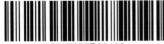

Made in the USA
Lexington, KY
07 August 2017